THE
INTERNET
FOR
PHYSICIANS
THIRD EDITION

With 93 Illustrations

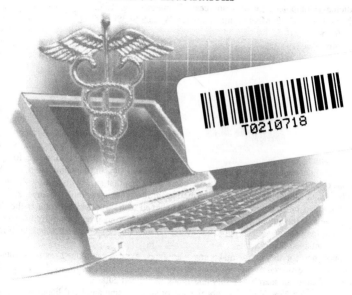

ROGER P. SMITH, M.D.
University of Missouri–Kansas City School of Medicine
Kansas City, Missouri
USA

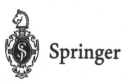

Springer

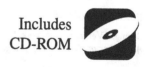

Includes
CD-ROM

Roger P. Smith, M.D.
Professor, Department of Obstetrics
    and Gynecology
Vice Chair and Program Director
University of Missouri–Kansas City
    School of Medicine
Kansas City, MO 64108
USA
bgumalley@earthlink.net

Library of Congress Cataloging-in-Publication Data
Smith, Roger P. (Roger Perry), 1949–
    The Internet for physicians / Roger P. Smith.—3rd ed.
        p.   cm.
    Includes bibliographical references and index.
    Additional material to this book can be downloaded from http://extras.springer.com.
    ISBN 0-387-95312-4 (s/c : alk. paper)

    1. Medicine—Computer network resources.   2. Internet.   I. Title.
    [DNLM: 1. Internet.   2. Medical Informatics.   W 26.5 S658i   2001]
    R859.7.D36 S54   2001
    004.67′8′02461—dc21   2001032809

Printed on acid-free paper.

Production managed by MaryAnn Brickner; manufacturing supervised by Joe Quatela.
Photocomposed copy prepared from the author's Microsoft Word files.
Printed and bound by Maple-Vail Book Manufacturing Group, York, PA.
Printed in the United States of America.

9 8 7 6 5 4 3 2 1

ISBN 0-387-95312-4   SPIN 10841220

Springer-Verlag   New York Berlin Heidelberg
A member of BertelsmannSpringer Science+Business Media GmbH

Preface to the Third Edition

In only a matter of months, the computer went from a device that dealt with information contained internally to a communication device. We have moved from manipulating data that we directly possess to borrowing information from locations we can't even identify, all because of the extraordinary growth and adoption of the Internet. What was once the province of propeller heads and pocket protector-toting computer "geeks," is now a staple in kindergarten classrooms and trendy coffee shops. We have gone from thinking a URL was a form of alien presence, to viewing it as natural footnote to bus advertising.

Like the Internet itself, interest in computing (both local and distant) has grown exponentially. When the first edition of this book was published, it was mainly the technophile fringe that was "surfing." Now grandmothers send e-mails to their stockbrokers, meals are planned and the groceries purchased across the Web, music videos can be previewed or concert tickets purchased—all with the help of the Internet. When our children come home from school, they are as likely to sign on to the Internet as they are to turn on the television. The Internet is a truly universal commodity. It seems everybody needs to be connected to the Web, just as they all seem to need to make cell-phone calls while changing lanes in heavy traffic.

This rapid and fundamental change in the role of the Internet has resulted in three very different editions of this text. The first edition attempted to introduce the concept of information transfer and communication and point the way toward a tool of the future. The second edition attempted to assuage trepidation in the use of this emerging tool and suggest the why and wherefore of being connected. The needs that drove those goals have almost completely disappeared. As a result, the bulk of the is edition can be more focused on the medical aspects of the Internet and its use, and much less on the nuts and bolts of connecting and communication through the Web.

Again in this edition, I hope to pique your curiosity and give you the adroitness and confidence to pursue the excitement of discovery. Be forewarned that the Internet is addictive: small doses give pleasure, leading to a desire for more; larger doses result in euphoria, loss of social contacts, and an enormous telephone bill. Don't blame me, it just happens. I just hope to get you involved in the habit.

Enjoy!

Roger P. Smith, M.D.
Kansas City, Missouri

Acknowledgments

The author is deeply indebted to the folks at Springer-Verlag, New York, for their encouragement, support, and technical expertise. Deserving of special thanks are Laura Gillan, the editor, cheerleader, and critic; Michelle Schmidt, a dedicated Web surfer who has tirelessly verified the validity of the Web sites listed in Appendix II, and MaryAnn Brickner, who has kept the format and look of the finished product something we can all be proud of. The author is also indebted to his tolerant family, and to the electronics industry for making it possible to do word processing in airports.

Roger P. Smith, M.D.
Kansas City, Missouri

Contents

1
The Web

We sell information. That is what we do in medicine. That is what we have always done. Today the difference is that we do it in an age of information. Information, medical and otherwise, is all around us. From pocket pagers that deliver stock quotes and sports scores to pocket digital assistants that wirelessly connect to the Internet, information is achieving the status of oxygen[1]—it is all around us and invisible. Today, information is managed, moved, and organized in ways never thought of in the past and will soon be managed in ways not yet conceived. In medicine, information is vital, but the exponential growth of knowledge available requires new approaches to its dissemination, access, and use. Central to this is the Internet. Information is now the province of anyone with a computer. This has led to "disintermediation": the ability of consumers to go directly to the source of information (or goods and services) directly, bypassing the intermediate steps of providers.

The Internet is nothing less than a library card to the world! One moment you can be browsing through the Library of Congress or looking at pictures from the National Library of Medicine and the next moment conversing with a colleague in Indonesia. At the most basic level, the Internet is a high-speed Web of worldwide computer-based information resources connected together. It is often defined as a network of computer networks. From its beginnings as a method of linking up 13 universities to allow the high-speed transfer of research data, the Internet has evolved to a system of millions of sites (computers) connected throughout the world. At the time of this writing, the Internet gains the equivalent of the entire population of Great Britain each month as new users. It has been estimated that in the United States, 8% of all the electricity generated goes to power the Internet, the computers connected to it, and the associated

---

[1] Oxygen is also the name of a computing project at the Massachusetts Institute of Technology that is aimed at achieving this goal.

hardware. According to the American Internet User Survey, more than 41.5 million adults in the United States are actively using the Internet. Of these Web users, 51% use the Web on a daily basis. The Internet auction service eBay will mediate over $7 billion in sales between its more than 22 million users during 2001.

Because the Internet is an invisible infrastructure of electronic links (like the telephone system), there is no master list of what information or resources are available or where! This is actually an advantage. Because there is no overall structure, the shape and face of the Internet are constantly changing to meet the needs of those who use it. Unlike the telephone system, which is planned and managed by a handful of readily identifiable organizations, the Internet has no corporate body. Rather, it is made up of loose associations of individuals, institutions, and corporations. As a result, the character of the Internet, indeed one of its founding premises, is that of change. Even in the catalog of sites listed in this book (Appendix 2), there are entries whose location has changed from the time we wrote about them to the time you try them.

The real power of the Internet is in the people and information that all those computers connect. The Internet is really a community that allows millions of people around the world to communicate with one another. People voluntarily share their time, ideas, and products, for the most part without any personal or financial gain. Although it is the computers that move the information around and execute the programs that allow us to access the information, it is the information itself and the people connected to the information that make the Internet useful!

What It Is and Where It Came From

The need to transfer information between computers was recognized soon after computers were developed. At first (the early 1960s), this type of information transfer was done with magnetic tapes or punch cards. These were then physically carried to the other computer to be used. Computer scientists then began exploring ways to directly connect remote computers and their users.

In 1969 the U.S. Department of Defense Advanced Research Projects Agency (ARPA) funded an experimental network called ARPANET. The main goal of the ARPANET research was to link together the Department of Defense and military research contractors (which included the University California at Santa Barbara and the University of California at Los Angeles, SRI International, and the University of Utah) and to develop a reliable network (Fig. 1.1). A "reliable network" involved the concept of dynamic rerouting. Dynamic rerouting, from the military perspective, allows communications on a network to be rerouted if part of the network is destroyed by an enemy attack.

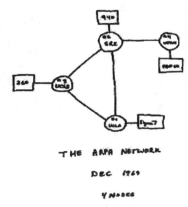

Figure 1.1. The original structure of the ARPANET as outlined in December 1969. (**http://www.computerhistory.org/timeline/topics/networks.page**)

Figure 1.2 demonstrates the idea of dynamic rerouting. Assume there are normally direct communication links between all four locations, A, B, C, and D. In Figure 1.1, the direct link between locations A and B has been severed (more likely by a backhoe than by hostile action). A and B cannot communicate directly along the dotted line. However, A can still send messages to B in a number of different ways, as indicated by the solid lines in the figure. For example, the message could be routed from A to D and then to B or from A to C and then to B or from A to D to C and then to B. On the Internet, there is always more than one way for the message to move from you to its intended recipient.

To accommodate the growing number of sites, the network had to be able to add and remove new sites easily and to allow computers of many different types to communicate effortlessly. This led to the development of the TCP/IP network protocol. TCP/IP (Transmission Control Protocol/Internet Protocol) is the language used by computers connected to the Internet to talk to each other. From the mid-1980s on, several physical networks were developed as increasing demands forced successive refinements and expansion.

Today, a number of suppliers maintain network backbones such as ANS Communications, AT&T, Compuserve, DIGEX, GTE Internetworking/ BBNPlanet, IBM Global Network, PSINet, Sprint IP Services, UUNET, and others. As a result, when we refer to "the Internet" we are not referring to a single set of wires or paths any more than there is a single telephone system that links the United States or the world. Each of the component networks are interconnected at various points by routers that pass the packets of information traveling the Web back and forth until they reach their destination computer.

In 1993, the World Wide Web (Web or WWW) was introduced and dramatically changed the face of computing. The Web, like Usenet and other networks, is just a portion of the Internet. The difference is that information on the Web is presented graphically using a standardized language that allows images, sound, and video information to be accessed and displayed graphically without knowledge of computer commands (those are taken care of for you by the Web browser).

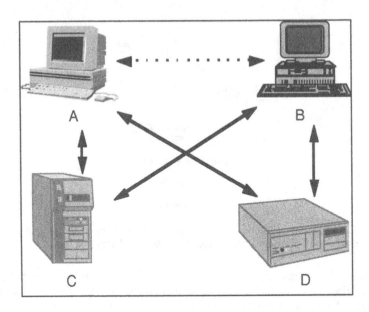

Figure 1.2. Dynamic rerouting allows multiple pathway for information transmission.

In many countries, the "backbone" of the Internet is funded by government organizations. In the United States, the National Science Foundation (NSF) currently funds such a backbone. To provide universities and research centers with remote access to supercomputer centers, the NSF funded a backbone network (NSFNET) that connects these centers. NSF also provided the funding for connections to the backbone for regional networks.

What It Can Do

Despite what your children may tell you, not everything is better on "The Net" and there really is life as we know it in homes and offices that are not connected. Despite this, approximately 40% of North Americans have access to the Web. The Internet is full of contradictions: it is blindingly fast and agonizingly slow, it is a loose confederation but works more reliably that systems that are tightly controlled, it is elegant and crass, it is public yet carries one of the most secure methods of communication available to the general public. Material that is vital to commerce mingles with sophomoric humor, and fine art passes smut in the electronic ether. It is these very contradictions that make surfing so compelling to many users.

A decision to connect to the Internet must be based on your needs and those of your family or office. It will be based on your practice style, volume, and personal needs. The uses of a small office will be different from those of a large multispecialty group; those of your grade school children will be different from those of a college student, and so on. One word of warning: the Internet is addictive. It is easy to lose track of time while surfing. Simple tasks such as reading e-mail can be accomplished in a matter of minutes; exploring all the Web has to offer cannot be completed. Like television, fishing, needlepoint, or other hobbies, some limits should be set.

Electronic Mail

Electronic mail was the first Internet application and is still the most popular one. E-mail is not limited to the Internet; e-mail messages can be moved through local or organizational networks, or through gateways to other networks and systems, such as CompuServe or America Online (AOL). Many, if not most, organizations have an internal e-mail system allowing rapid and open communications within the organization and, via outside connections, communications to organizations and individuals anywhere computer networks reach. Your hospital or university may be willing to provide e-mail services to you at no cost.

Goods and Services

The fastest-growing segment of the Internet is business. Full-scale Internet showrooms allow you to do everything but touch the merchandise; virtual reality movies allow you to look at an item in three dimensions, move it about, listen to it, change its color, get technical information, and ask questions—all without a salesperson hovering near. You may purchase items directly using credit cards (directly, by e-mail or telephone confirmation) and have them shipped overnight to arrive the next morning. You can even send "virtual flowers" (a bouquet of flowers with your personal message that arrives by electronic mail or directions to a special Web site) when you miss a special event.

Remote Presence

Remote presence at one time meant the ability to work on a computer from a distance just as if you were actually sitting at the keyboard of that machine. The Internet now allows remote presence to include such things as video conferencing and telemedicine. Whether it is checking a cardiogram, consulting on a radiograph, or evaluating fetal heart tones, the Internet is almost the next best thing to being there.

Patient Care

Patient care has been (or may be) enhanced through the use of the Internet. Patient records may be sent or retrieved (with appropriate privacy controls) by way of the Internet, allowing labor rooms to have the most recent prenatal records, or surgeons to have the biopsy report from an out-of-state hospital. Drug interactions may be checked, the most recent journal article may be scanned, or a consultation with a distant colleague may be completed by connections to the Internet. Patients can get information (both authoritative and otherwise) on their condition, treatment, and alternatives via Internet sites.

Information Retrieval

Information can take many forms: from the traditional, such as the response to a query about a patient's blood count, to pictures, sound, or video images. Information on the Internet resides in many places and forms. When you are connected to the Internet you can access these repositories in many ways.

Database Searching

In the same way that you conduct a database search in a hospital or university library using a card catalog (if your library still has one) or CD-ROM technology, you can search databases through the Internet. You can access many of the same databases, such as MedLine, Toxline, CINAHL, and others just as you would through your library but without having to go to the library and wait your turn. The Internet also allows you to search resources anywhere on the globe with the same ease as you would in your local library. A specialized version of database searching occurs when you ask the hospital computer for a patient's laboratory results. In many locations, even these data (with suitable security controls) may be accessed from remote locations, through (you guessed it) the Internet.

Remote File Access

When computer users give their permission, files placed in their computer's storage device (generally a hard drive or other mass storage device) may be accessed by others connected through the Internet. This ability to "download" (take from) or "upload" (give to) files from one computer to another allows users access to the latest versions of information. If you have set up your home computer to allow such transfers (and it is turned on), you can access your own files from a hotel room anywhere in the world. (OK, it does have to have a telephone line, you have to have a computer that can talk on the telephone, you have to have access to an Internet service providers, etc., but you get the idea.)

2
Connecting and Communicating on the Web

Unlike with telephone in the era of AT&T or today's cable television, there is no primary local provider or standardized hardware to fall back on. To connect and communicate on the Web you will need some basic computer hardware (much of which you may already have) and a method of making the electronic connection. The choices of how, with what, and with whom are the next issues we need to address.

Getting Connected

There are four basic ways to connect to the Internet: make a direct connection over dedicated communications lines, use your computer to connect to a university or hospital computer system that has "Internet access buy time" and connections from a commercial Internet service provider, or use an indirect service provider.

Direct Connection to the Internet

A direct or dedicated connection wires your computer directly to the Internet through a dedicated machine called a router or gateway. The connection is made over a special kind of telephone line (T3, T1, or ISDN line). The gateway makes you an "official" Internet computer that must remain on-line at all times. This type of direct connection is very expensive to install and maintain. For this reason, it is usually used only by large companies or institutions rather than by individuals or small businesses. This type of connection (and the need to be continuously connected to the network) potentially leaves the files on your computer open to inspection, theft, or alteration by hackers. This same consideration can happen if you choose to connect by way of a (TV) cable modem (see below), which leaves you connected on a continuous basis. To counteract this possibility, systems of this type should be protected by firewall software, which detects and prevents suspicious activities.

Connecting Through Another's Gateway

Another way to connect to the Internet is to use a gateway that another company or institution has established. In this case, a company, university, or hospital that has an Internet gateway allows you to connect to the Internet using their system. The connection is usually made through a modem or remote terminal. Many hospitals and health services organizations allow staff access to the Internet through the institution's facilities. The only disadvantage is that the institution may not offer full Internet access, but only e-mail and newsgroup facilities. To use an institution's access, you will need proper identification: a login ID and password. The information services or computer services department is the place to inquire about getting access and authorization. For the individual, this is the best type of access to have if full Internet access is available. Someone other than you maintains the computer system and the Internet connection and, most importantly, pays for the connection.

Connecting Through a Commercial Service Provider

Connecting to the Internet through a service provider is much the same process as using another's gateway. The service provider builds and maintains the gateway and sells Internet connection access to individuals and small companies. There are many different types of services available through commercial providers. Service providers usually charge a flat fee for membership and for a certain number of hours of Internet access per month. Some providers also charge based on the amount of extra time you spend connected to the Net or on the amount and size of e-mail messages that you send. Plans that offer unlimited access are more common now, though without the time pressure to limit your surfing you may find yourself missing major holidays and anniversaries.

Service providers may provide you with a SLIP (Serial Line Internet Protocol) or PPP (Point-to-Point Protocol) connection. With this type of connection, you dial in to the service provider's computer and connect through the gateway. Your computer, as long as it stays connected, becomes an "official" part of the Internet. With a SLIP or PPP connection, you have full Internet access, up to the power and storage capacity of your own computer. The major disadvantage of using a SLIP or PPP connection is the amount of technical computer expertise that is usually required to install and maintain this type of connection on your computer.

It is now most common to find Internet service providers who offer PPP connections by modem. These services usually provide only access, though an e-mail account may be included. Most offer the convenience of a local telephone number and graduated fee structures that allow you to choose the level of service that fits your needs and usage patterns. Many newer Internet browsers include setup or installation software that smooths out the old problems of installation and sign-on. For many users, this has become the preferred method of connection.

Connecting Through an Indirect Service Provider

On-line value-added services such as America Online, CompuServe, Delphi, and Prodigy supply their own content in addition to Internet access in varying degrees. The advantage again is that the inner workings of connecting to the Internet are hidden to the user, so connecting is a simple process. Some of the disadvantages are that unrestricted Internet access is not available through all on-line providers, and on-line services fees often include not only a membership fee but also connect time charges. If you are going to use the Internet for only two to three hours per month, or want to take advantage of the other services offered, this might be an alternative to consider as a starting place. If you don't need the support these services provide, most of the same content is now available directly on the Internet.

Hardware

If you have access to a telephone line (or cable TV), a modem, and a computer, you can connect to the Internet. The hardware needed to become a part of the family of Internet users is relatively simple and inexpensive. Of course, you can add on features such as faster processing, more memory, or chrome curb feelers that run the price up quite a bit. For this discussion we will review the basics and leave the flourishes up to you.

Dedicated Hardware

Several new options for dedicated or semi-dedicated Internet access have become available. Set-top boxes (WebTV) are roughly the size of a small video recorder and are designed to connect to your television in much the same way. The set-top box must also be connected to a telephone line. These devices send your request for Internet information to a provider (usually restricted to the maker of the box) and the results of that request are sent down either the phone line or the cable TV connection and displayed on the screen. These devices are priced in the range of $300 and require a service contract with the provider of approximately $20 per month. Speed is generally acceptable, but the resolution of a television set is much less than that of a computer monitor, limiting the amount and clarity of the information presented. As a dedicated system, these boxes cannot perform any other computer functions. This system may be best suited for those on a tight budget who need access only to text and e-mail.

Specialized Computers and Devices

The introduction of specialized Web computers has changed Internet access. Computer systems such as the I-Mac bridge the gap between dedicated Web devices and the more general computers discussed below. These devices allow most, if not all, general computer functionality while retaining the ease of connection and setup, along with economies of price, of the specialized devices.

Another subset of specialized Internet computers are the popular pocket digital assistants such as the Palm Pilot, Handspring, and others. Many of these devices have the ability to connect to the Internet by wire or by wireless means. These computers have specialized programs for tracking appointments, telephone and personal contacts, expenses, and other functions. Some cellular telephones available now, or in the near future, offer a form of limited Internet access and must be considered a specialized form of computing devise. Availability of services, restrictions on screen size and capabilities, and data transmission speeds currently limit this mode of access, but evolving technologies promise to change these limitations.

General Computers

A more general and versatile solution to Internet access is a general-purpose computer. Even dedicated Internet nerds occasionally have to write a letter or a check, do homework, or play a game. By using a general-purpose computer for your Internet connection, you have the flexibility to function independently of the Internet.

IBM vs. Mac;—A Matter of Religion

While it is heresy for a Macintosh user to admit, both systems work fine. The differences between the systems have narrowed and it is really a matter of personal preference. The one notable difference is the I-Mac, which is designed to be a true "plug-and-play" Internet system while retaining the capabilities of a more general computer. Often the choice between one system and the other is based on maintaining similarity between a new and an old system, the system at the office or hospital, or (better still) that of a knowledgeable friend to whom you turn for help or advice. (Compatibility with children at college or living away from home may also be desirable, although asking them for advice may be out of the question.)

Desktop vs. Laptop

The next hardware decision to be made is where and how the computer will be used. If the computer will stay put at home or the office, a desktop model will be the best choice. These have the greatest flexibility, and offer the most computing power for the price. Portable units (laptops) allow you to take your computing power with you when you travel. (This chapter is being written in a hotel room, for example.) These units are smaller, but often roughly three times more expensive than a similar desktop unit. Only your anticipated usage can determine which is best for you.

Memory, Speed, Peripherals, and All That

If your main use for the computer will be Internet access, simple word processing, and household applications such as balancing a checkbook, last year's computer model will be sufficient. Processor speed is generally less important that the amount of memory (RAM) available in determining the speed of Internet applications. New or old, the machine should probably have 32 MB (megabytes) of memory or more. Internet browsers use part of the computer's hard disk to store temporary information, and Internet files, especially those with images, can take up vast amounts of memory. Consequently, a moderate amount of space on a hard disk or removable high-density cartridge or floppy system (like a Zip drive) is a necessity. A gigabyte (GB, roughly 1,000 megabytes) is probably the starting point for today's systems, with 4 to 8 GB or more desirable, readily available, and very affordable.

If you have or are buying an older computer for Internet access, make sure that it is compatible with today's high-speed modems. If you plan to use a cable modem (see below) or your hospital's Ethernet (high-speed internal network connection), you should be sure that your computer either has direct Ethernet connections or can accept a circuit board ("card") that will give you that capability. In general, old Macintoshes tend to be more suitable than old IBM compatibles, but check the specifics before you decide to buy or trade up.

You will want a color monitor for your computer, but unless you will be doing specialized applications, the generic color monitor often sold with computers will be adequate. You will probably want a printer so you can make hard copies of e-mail or other information you find on the Web. Almost all modern printers can handle graphics, so the only real decision is color versus black and white. This is a personal preference (and budget) decision. Lastly, you will want external speakers for your computer, especially if it is an IBM type. While optional, many Web sites now contain voice or music that are greatly enhanced by bringing the sound out of actual speakers instead of the muffled world of bits and bytes.

Speaking to the Outside World

One part of the hardware decisions to be made is how you will connect your computer to the Web itself. If you are lucky enough to be able to connect your computer to the information system of a larger hospital or university, you can take advantage of high-speed connections directly through the use of a network card installed within the computer or an Ethernet port. From home, the most common method is to use existing or dedicated telephone lines and the computer equivalent of a telephone, the modem.

Modems allow your computer to convert the digital information it uses internally into an analog signal (like voice) that the telephone system usually handles, and vice versa. Modems come in various types but all communicate at a selection of set speeds that determine the amount of information transferred per second, measured in bauds. Like many things in life, the faster the better. A higher speed modem can make the difference between receiving your sports scores as the game ends and getting them after the morning paper has already given them to you. In today's market, the effective starting speed for a modem is 56,000 bps (bits per second, 56 KB or kilobaud). Standard modems are available in three forms: internal (to be mounted inside the computer box itself), external (attached to the computer by cables but located outside in its own enclosure), and PCMIA or PC card (a fat credit card-sized device used with laptop computers). The choice of internal or external is one of purely personal preference; internal modems must match the computer type and model, while external ones are more universal and can be moved from one computer to another if you change machines.

Wireless modems are devices that allow you to connect to an Internet service provider through the same network that handles cellular telephone calls. The type of cellular network you use and the availability of a suitable service provider limits this option to a few large metropolitan areas. The amount of information that can be downloaded and viewed is limited by both the device usually used (palm-top computers or the newer versions of hybrid cellular telephones) and the speed of the connection. Consequently, this option is of inadequate utility for all but a few specialized users.

The same coaxial cable that brings cable television into your office or home can send information out at speeds of up to 1.5 million bits per second. Several companies offer special devices (and services) to connect your computer directly to the cable lines. These special cable modems can improve performance, but that performance may degrade as more users in your neighborhood connect to this party line. Internet cable connections do not interfere with your television reception and prevent tying up a telephone line, but the connection is generally more expensive than the usual modem connection options (generally two to three times more expensive). Cable modems generally remain turned on at all times because it may take as long as 15 minutes for the modem to synchronize itself with the rest of the system when it is first turned on. Some cable systems will provide a telephone number for access when you travel but this is not automatically the case (and will be at normal telephone connection speeds). Many cable companies restrict the use of cable modems to personal use only, so you may have to make special arrangements if you are going to connect your office or home business to the system. The continuous nature of the cable connection can potentially open you to security concerns (as discussed further below).

In some areas, an emerging hybrid between satellite and modem connections is available. In this system, your computer requests information from a distant computer using a high-speed telephone modem. The information returns to your computer through an ultra-high-speed link using the same digital satellite system that brings television signals in to your home. Since the bulk of information transferred is to your computer, rather than from it, this system provides very rapid display of the requested information. This hybrid is currently available on a limited basis and will improve service only if you do not need to transmit many blocks of information yourself. (That is, it is best suited to home use, not for commercial or business applications.)

Software

To access the Web, you will need a Web browser program (agent) on either your computer or your service provider's. The most popular programs of this type are Netscape Navigator or Communicator and Microsoft Internet Explorer. (Also see a discussion of metabrowsers in Chapter 3.) A Web browser program interprets and displays the hypertext documents that it finds on the Web. Either through their own programming or the use of specialized small plug-in programs, browsers also have the ability to play music, display moving images, supply portals for interactive sound and video, and perform many other functions beyond simple hypertext links. These browsers make navigating the Web easy and intuitive; the hypertext links are highlighted and you simply "point and click" with your mouse.

Located near the top of the browser window is a series of buttons that assist with the display of information. The appearance of these buttons varies slightly from browser to browser (Fig. 2.1) and can be modified in the program's preference file. The "back" and "forward" buttons display information from a list of places you have been during the current surfing session. This is possible because the program keeps a running list of the information requested (see below). This allows you to explore an idea and then backtrack to go off in another direction.

Buttons offer options to "reload" or "refresh" the information displayed (either the entire page or just the images present). Pressing reload causes the browser to re-request the entire document and freshly display the results. This may be desirable if errors of transmission result in missing or uninter-

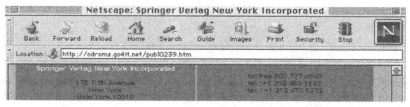

Figure 2.1. Buttons located near the top of the browser window make navigation easier.

pretable data. Because the browser often stores copies of Web pages to make the display process faster, pressing reload can provide an updated version of rapidly changing data. Examples might include following an on-line antique auction or the fluctuations of the stock market.

As might be expected, the "Print" button results in a copy of the information displayed being sent to the printer. If no printer is available or specified, an error message or worse is encountered. The edit and search buttons allow you to work with the commands that display the screen or to find a word or phrase within the displayed information. This search is NOT the same as searching for information on the Web itself. These last two buttons will not be used by most surfers.

Most Web browsers have a "home page" that opens when the program is begun or when the navigation "home" button is pressed. This is actually a special Web site provided by the maker of the Web browser (Fig. 2.2), but it may be changed by the user to any Internet site you wish. All Web sites have a welcome page, the index or home page that you see when you first connect to that site. This home page may just give the name of the site but usually it contains a list of resources and links available at the site. Almost any Internet site may be designated as the home page for your browser. You may wish to have the browser display stock quotes, a vacation site, or a personal Web page when it opens. The home page may be recalled at any time by pressing the "Home" button.

Located below the buttons on the browser screen there is a box that contains the address of the site being displayed. This is the made up of the URL for the host computer, combined with information about the specific page or file that is

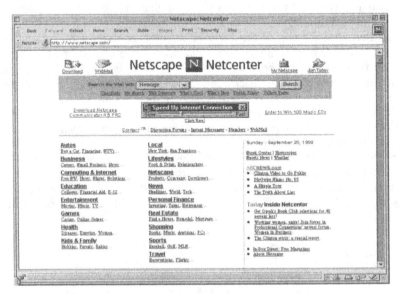

Figure 2.2. Most Web browsers provide or allow the user to specify a "home page" to which the browser returns every time the program is begun. In this example, it is the opening screen from Netscape communicator.

to be displayed appended as a series of information separated by slashes. As noted earlier, this series tells the browser and host computer what form to use transmitting the data and the type of data that is expected. You may enter the URL for an Internet site directly to obtain its data. Most browsers will also allow you to enter just the organization's name, such as **Sony** or **NBC**, and the browser will fill in the **http://www.** and the **.com**. This shorthand is convenient but it only works if the organization is in the zone "com" and uses the World Wide Web (www).

Providers

There are several basic questions you should ask when you consider getting access to the Internet through a provider. First, what kind of computer do you have to work with? While most providers support a variety of computer types, from PC and Macintosh to minicomputers and mainframes, the technical capabilities are more important than the brand name. The processing power, speed, and storage capacity of your computer are important. Be sure to have this type of technical information ready when you contact a service provider.

Second, what is your own level of technical knowledge and comfort when working with your computer? It is important to understand that there are many links to this connection chain. As a result, you may have to become involved in levels of technical details that you did not anticipate. Some Internet providers, for a fee, will help you install the connection software on your computer and get it working, removing most of the need for technical expertise.

Third, is there a provider with a local telephone number that you can use to connect? Some providers advertise 1-800 numbers that you use, although the additional cost of these lines is often buried in the charges these providers make. The point here is to avoid additional telephone charges. Without a local number, you will be paying additional costs to your telephone company. If you travel frequently, a national provider may offer local telephone contacts in major cities, also removing the need for long-distance charges.

Fourth, what set of Internet services or tools does the provider offer? You may be perfectly satisfied with just an e-mail account, but it is unlikely. Be sure to check the details of what is offered and what, if any, additional charges there might be for items such as the number of e-mail messages sent or the use of space for your own Web page. Ask about the ability to add additional services in the future if you decide that you need them. Some providers impose inappropriately high service fees to change your service once it has been established. You may also wish to inquire about the availability of service packages that result in net savings.

Fifth, what is the cost of this connection? Be sure that all the restrictions and assumptions are fully identified. One provider offered unlimited access to the Internet for a very low monthly charge. The hitch was that you were allowed to be connected for a maximum of only 90 minutes in one stretch. After that, you

Table 2.1. Examples of common questions for Internet providers

Computer compatibility / hardware needs	Can I use any computer to access the service?
	Do you support all computer brands and operating systems? If not, which?
	How powerful does the computer have to be?
	How fast can my Modem be?
Software	Who installs the software?
	Is the software specific to the provider, or may I use recognized browsers such as Netscape or Internet Explorer?
	Who provides technical support for the software? Are they available? When? How?
Access	Is the access point local?
	Are there local access points if I travel?
	Are there phone related charges involved?
	Is access restricted as to time of day, duration of use, frequency of use, etc.?
Fees	What is the base cost of service? Are there packages that save money?
	What generates extra charges? How much?
	Can I upgrade as needed? (New features? Faster connections?)

were automatically disconnected. Of course, you could immediately try to dial back in, but.... This may be perfectly satisfactory for an infrequent e-mail user, but for someone trying to search the Net for information 90 minutes goes by very quickly.

Last, what kind of technical support does the provider offer? Always be an informed buyer. If a provider does not have the time or desire to answer your questions before you buy, think about the kind of support you are likely to get when something goes wrong. If you have trouble coping now when your computer gives you fits, ask some tough questions about the kind and level of support from the provider. Also ask about the support schedule of the provider (e.g., 24 hours a day, business hours only, etc.). There are enough providers that you should be able to find one that actually values your business. Table 2.1 offers a partial list of questions you might consider when interviewing a perspective provider.

Information Transfer

Connecting to the Internet is only the first step in exploring the information contained in all those computers all over the world. The Internet is not only for getting mail and looking up airline flight schedules. To take full advantage of all the Internet has to offer, it make sense to become acquainted with what is out there, how the information is passed along, and the tools that are used to request and display the data.

Internet Addresses

Every computer that is on the Internet is given a unique address, just as each telephone user has a unique combination of area code and telephone number. Even if you sign on only occasionally, you have an address, even if it is only temporarily assigned (on loan) from your Internet service provider. Once you know other users' Internet addresses, you can send mail, transfer files, look at their Web pages, and even have a conversation.

Internet address consist of four numbers (0–255) separated by periods:

206.136.111.252

This address makes sense to the routers and computers attached to the system, but is not very convenient for human users. For this reason, domain names or universal locator codes (URLs) are used. The individual user chooses names on the Internet that are registered with a central registry (InterNIC in the United States) to avoid conflicts. When a Web browser attempts to contact a distant computer, Internet routers look up this number in a table of computer addresses and uses the number to pass the message along. This is normally invisible to the user, but occasionally a message such as "No DNS entry exists" will be seen. This occurs infrequently and may be caused by something as simple as a minor misspelling of the domain name. (This is different from the "404 File Not Found" message that means that the distant computer was found but not the specific page of information.)

All Internet addresses follow the same format as shown in Figure 2.3. Examples of an Internet domain name are

www.umkc.edu
www.isd.umkc.edu

If the optional geographic zone is included, these could also be written as

www.umkc.edu.us
www.isd.umkc.edu.us

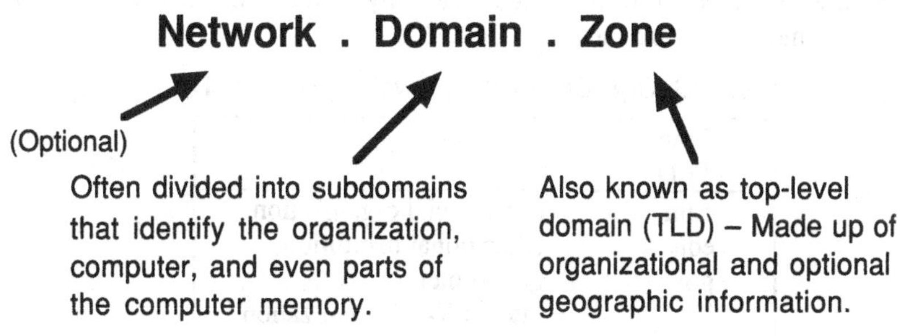

Network . Domain . Zone

(Optional)

Often divided into subdomains that identify the organization, computer, and even parts of the computer memory.

Also known as top-level domain (TLD) – Made up of organizational and optional geographic information.

Figure 2.3. The structure of Internet domain names. (Spaces have been added before and after the periods for clarity; they are not a part of the address.)

Table 2.2. Examples of geographic top-level domains

Domain	Meaning
at	Austria
au	Australia
ca	Canada
ch	Switzerland ("Confoederatio Helvetia")
de	Germany ("Deutschland")
fr	France
gr	Greece
no	Norway
jp	Japan
sw.	Sweden
us	United States

The domain and zone in an address are often made up of subdomains, each one separated by a period. To understand an address name, read it from right to left. The rightmost section (the zone) is the most general, and the subdomains become more specific as you read to the left. In our example, the zone is made up of **edu** and **us**, and the domain is **isd.umkc** with the subdomains of **isd** and **umkc**. That rightmost entry is the zone or top-level domain, and there are two different sets of top-level domains (TLDs): organizational domains and the geographic domains.

In our example, **www.umkc.edu.us**, the geographic subdomain is **us**. That identifies the computer as being located in the United States (see Table 2.2 for other geographic designations). The next subdomain of the zone identifies the type of organization as educational institution, **edu**. The domain **umkc** identifies the actual organization, the University of Missouri—Kansas City. The set of organizational zones (TLD) was defined mostly for use in the United States (see Table 2.3).

Most Internet addresses you will encounter in browsing the Web will include prefixes and suffixes that tell the computer (yours and theirs) in what format to send the data and the type of data that is expected. This makes up the Universal Resource Locator (URL). The prefixes indicate the document type (protocol to use) and are separated from the domain name by a colon and two slashes (://). Typical document types are shown in Table 2.4.

Table 2.3. Organizational top-level domains (TLD)

Zone (TLD)	Meaning
com	commercial organization
edu	educational institution
gov	government
int	international organization
mil	military
net	networking organization
org	nonprofit organization

Many URL addresses include suffixes that indicate the pathname, which indicates the file and data type to be retrieved. The pathname is separated from the zone or TLD designation by a slash, and may itself contain additional slashes to indicate subdirectories or folders. The last portion of this pathname includes to type of file being referenced. These indicators are separated from the file name by a period. Typical data types are shown in Table 2.5.

Table 2.4. Examples of common document types

Prefix	Meaning
http	Hypertext (the Web)
https	Hypertext with a secure link
ftp	File transfer protocol
gopher	Gopher files
mailto	E-mail addresses

Table 2.5. Examples of suffixes that denote file type

Suffix	File type	Suffix	File type
.a	application/octet-stream	.mpeg	video/mpeg
.ai	application/postscript	.mpg	video/mpeg
.aif	audio/x-aiff	.ms	application/x-troff-ms
.aifc	audio/x-aiff	.mv	video/x-sgi-movie
.aiff	audio/x-aiff	.nc	application/x-netcdf
.arc	application/octet-stream	.o	application/octet-stream
.au	audio/basic	.oda	application/oda
.avi	application/x-troff-msvideo	.pbm	image/x-portable-bitmap
.bcpio	application/x-bcpio	.pdf	application/pdf
.bin	application/octet-stream	.pgm	image/x-portable-graymap
.c	text/plain	.pl	text/plain
.c++	text/plain	.pnm	image/x-portable-anymap
.cc	text/plain	.ppm	image/x-portable-pixmap
.cdf	application/x-netcdf	.ps	application/postscript
.cpio	application/x-cpio	.qt	video/quicktime
.djv	image/x-djvu	.ras	image/x-cmu-rast
.djvu	image/x-djvu	.rgb	image/x-rgb
.dump	application/octet-stream	.roff	application/x-troff
.dvi	application/x-dvi	.rtf	application/rtf
.eps	application/postscript	.rtx	application/rtf
.etx	text/x-setext	.saveme	application/octet-stream
.exe	application/octet-stream	.sh	application/x-shar
.gif	image/gif	.shar	application/x-shar
.gtar	application/x-gtar	.snd	audio/basic
.gz	application/octet-stream	.src	application/x-wais-source
.h	text/plain	.sv4cpio	application/x-sv4cpio
.hdf	application/x-hdf	.sv4crc	application/x-sv4crc
.hqx	application/octet-stream	.t	application/x-troff
.htm	text/html	.tar	application/x-tar
.html	text/html	.tex	application/x-tex
.iw4	image/x-iw44	.texi	application/x-texinfo
.iw44	image/x-iw44	.texinfo	application/x-texinfo
.ief	image/ief	.text	text/plain
.java	text/plain	.tif	image/tiff
.jfif	image/jpeg	.tiff	image/tiff

Table 2.5. Examples of suffixes that denote file type

.jfif-tbnl	image/jpeg	.tr	application/x-troff
.jpe	image/jpeg	.tsv	text/tab-separated-values
.jpeg	image/jpeg	.txt	text/plain
.jpg	image/jpeg	.ustar	application/x-ustar
.latex	application/x-latex	.uu	application/octet-stream
.man	application/x-troff-man	.wav	audio/x-wav
.me	application/x-troff-me	.wsrc	application/x-wais-source
.mime	message/rfc822	.xbm	image/x-xbitmap
.mov	video/quicktime	.xpm	image/x-xpixmap
.movie	video/x-sgi-movie	.xwd	image/x-xwindowdump
.mpe	video/mpeg	.z	application/octet-stream

As a rule, Internet addresses are case sensitive: If you see an address with some uppercase letters, it is not safe to change them to lowercase.

For electronic mail the structure is only slightly different: the person's user ID followed by the @ symbol, followed by the unique name of the computer host (the domain name) but omitting the final pathname. Therefore, every e-mail address always has two parts, the user ID and the domain, put together like this:

userid@domain

FTP and HTML

FTP (File Transfer Protocol) is technically the set of specifications that specify the way Internet file transfer works. Practically, however, FTP is used to refer to a service that allows you to copy a file from any Internet host to another Internet host (usually your computer). Therefore, FTP is another example of an Internet application that allows you to access a remote host computer. FTP only allows you to look at the file names on a remote computer and then copy (download) them to your computer. On some remote sites, you can also upload to the host computer, but you cannot "work" on the remote host. FTP is one of the most widely used Internet services. FTP allows you to "fetch" files, leading to the common name for one FTP program, Fetch. FTP protocols are also the ones used when you request software upgrades, samples, or purchase software directly over the Internet from a provider's Web page.

Many of the available Windows-based and all of the Macintosh-based Internet programs allow you to use FTP with a simple "point and click" and make the whole process easy. A typical FTP inquiry is shown in Figure 2.4.

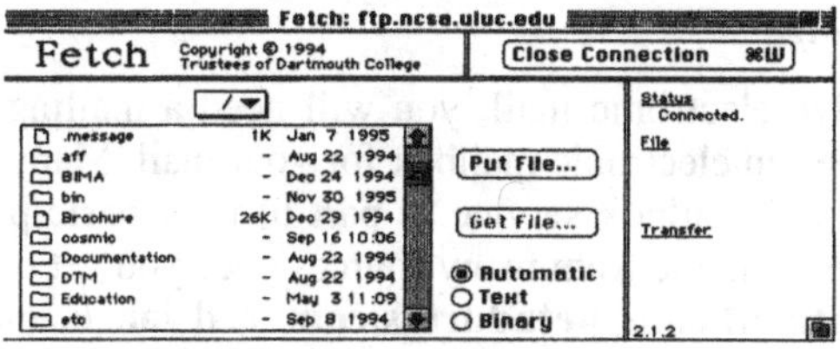

Figure 2.4. The screen of a typical FTP inquiry made using the Fetch program shows the elements common to all FTP sessions: a list of directories and files that may be downloaded, but without much additional information to indicate the applicability or usefulness of the files for the task at hand.

Using the Web to Communicate

Today, the computer is used more as a communication device than as an information processor. Not long ago, all of the data that your computer used was housed within its physical case. Now, the majority of the information processed comes from some outside source. Whether you are communicating with patients, e-mailing a child at college, or submitting a manuscript (as in the case if this book itself), the ability of the computer to communicate has become one of its major functions.

E-mail

E-mail combines a word processor function and a "post office" function in one program: You type the message and identify the recipient's e-mail address and your return address (commonly supplied automatically by your communications software). Then you "send" your message. The electronic post office in your system takes over and passes your message on to the network with an appropriate set of electronic tags that tell the network(s) where to send the message.

Your message often will pass through a series of intermediate networks to reach the recipient's address. Because networks can and do use different e-mail formats, a gateway at each network translates the format of your e-mail message into one that the next network understands. Each gateway also reads the destination address of your message and sends the message on in the direction of the destination mailbox. The routing choice takes into consideration the size of your message and the amount of traffic on various networks. Because of this routing, the amount of time to send messages from you to the same person will vary: on one occasion, it might be only a few seconds, but on others, it might be a few hours.

When your message reaches its destination, the recipient can read the message, respond to you with just a few keystrokes, forward your message to someone else, file it, print it, or delete it.

Sending Your Message

To send and receive electronic mail, you will need a mailing program and a service that provides an electronic mailbox for your mail. Many Internet service providers offer e-mail mailbox service as part of their basic package and free e-mail accounts are available from many sources once you get on line. Examples are **juno.com, hotmail.com, netaddress.com**, and **yahoo.com**. (Advertising fees the companies charge offset the cost of this service; there is no charge to the user.)

To handle your messages you need a program such as Eudora (Lite or Pro), Juno, Outlook Express, GroupWise, Netscape (Communicator), Internet Explorer, or others. (Most are available for both the IBM and Macintosh environments.) All mailing programs share certain basic functionality: they all must find out who the message is for, what it is about, and what the information is you want sent as the message. (It need not be text, but may be files, images, sounds, video, or a combination of several types.)

Anatomy of an E-Mail Message

E-mail messages always have several features in common regardless of the program used to create the e-mail. A typical e-mail message includes a "From" line with the sender's electronic address, a date and time line, a "To" line with the recipient's electronic address, a "Subject" line, and the body of the message. In most mail programs the "From" is hidden in the outgoing message, but will be a part of the message when it is received on the other end. The "To" line indicates the address to which the message is sent. If the message is to be sent to several other people at the same time, their addresses will also appear on this line. If there are any spelling or punctuation mistakes in the recipient's address, the message will be sent back to you from the electronic post office indicating that it was undeliverable. (The message is said to "bounce back" when this happens.) If the message is being copied to others, their addresses will appear after "Copies to." Copying or forwarding messages to others is easy to do with most mail programs. For this reason, be very prudent in what you say in a message; it may go further than you expect.

The "Subject" line is the place to give a clear, one-line description of your message. This description is usually displayed when someone checks his or her e-mail. The "Subject" line tells the recipient the contents of the message. Its subject lines should be very clear because the description is often the basis for deciding what is read first and what may be discarded without opening.

Next comes the body of the message. While most e-mail messages are text, if your computer and the recipient's computer have the facilities, you can send data files, sound and visual images, computer programs, and even computer viruses via e-mail. Attach additional files sparingly. These can rapidly increase the size of your message, which results in slowdowns and delayed delivery. Not all recipients will have the computer power, memory, or appropriate programs to open and interpret these attachments, so be sure they are what the recipient wants or needs and not just so much digital junk.

Many mail programs can automatically attach a signature line at the end of your message. The signature line can include the sender's name, telephone number, postal address, and Internet address. Most programs that offer this will allow the user to turn this feature on and off as desired. Figure 2.5 contains sample e-mail messages. The format may vary on your system, but the general idea will be the same.

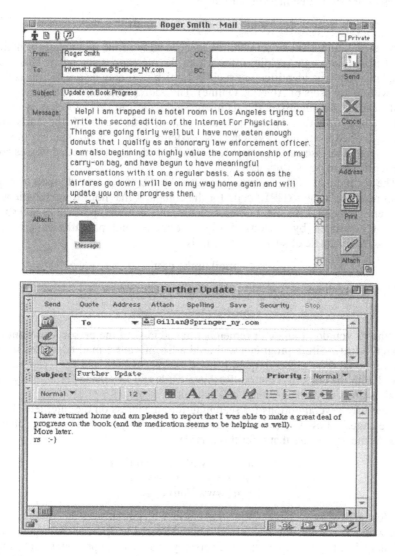

Figure 2.5. A sample E-mail message as sent from GroupWise (top) and Netscape Communicator (bottom).

Do You Have that Address Handy?

To send e-mail you must know the recipient's address; there is no "general delivery" or American Express office where you can leave messages. All e-mail addresses are structured in a similar manner:

mailboxname@hostname

All e-mail addresses begin with the identification of the individual (or mailbox if it is a corporate recipient) for whom the message is intended. This will often be an obvious identification such as **rsmith** or it may be cryptic (as is the case with many users of America Online). The address may also be a compound identification that identifies the recipient and some form of sub-classification such as **obgyn.rsmith**. When such a subclassification is used, the parts are always divided using a period. On most systems, case does not matter, though most e-mail addresses are in lower case. (URLs and other Internet addresses are case sensitive, so pay attention.)

The second part of the address, separated by the "@", is the domain or universal resource locator (URL) code for the computer that houses the recipient's mail service (host). Like other domain names, this is made up of zones and sub-domains separated by periods. Spaces, commas, and parentheses are not allowed. An example of such subdomains is:

mail.umkc.edu

Combining these parts results in the final e-mail address:

rsmith@mail.umkc.edu

What if you don't know or remember the address of the person you want to contact? Most mailing programs will hold a list of your e-mail addresses in an address book. You place frequently used addresses here and they can be retrieved with the click of a button. Business cards and letterheads often carry the e-mail address or you can always call and ask.

There are several options for searching for an address on the Internet. These "white pages" allow you to look up an address just as you would in a telephone book. Some of the sites that offer this service are:

http://www.swithchboard.com
http://www.whowhere.com
http://www.Four11.com

Most mail systems have a human overseer who administers the system. This (overworked) administrator will read mail addressed to "postmaster" (postmaster@domain). If you are sure that the person you are having problems contacting is likely to be a part of that domain, you can request help with the proper address to use. This is also the person to whom problems can be reported, but this should be limited to significant abuses or system failings, not just someone who doesn't open their mail often or has bad spelling.

Table 2.6. Common Internet abbreviations

Abbreviation	Meaning
AFAIK	As Far As I Know
AFK	Away From Keyboard
ADN	Any Day Now
BAK	Back At Keyboard
BTW	By The Way
FAQ	Frequently Asked Question
FWIW	For What It's Worth
FYI	For Your Information
GD&R	Grinning, Ducking, & Running
IMHO	In My Humble Opinion
IMO	In My Opinion
IOW	In Other Words
LOL	Laughing Out Loud
OTOH	On The Other Hand
ROFL	Rolling On the Floor Laughing
RSN	Real Soon Now
RTFM	Read The Funny Manual
RTM	Read The Manual
TIA	Thanks In Advance
WRT	With Respect To
YMMV	Your Mileage May Vary

Know the Code

There are several short cuts and conventions that make electronic mail more efficient and user friendly, but more arcane for the novice. For convenience, there are a number of widely used abbreviations found in Internet communications, including those shown in Table 2.6.

Although e-mail allows easy expression of ideas, it does not allow the recipient of your message to hear the tone of your voice or see the body language that accompanies your message. A bit of the impish nature of the Internet has arisen to help with this problem by the development of typed symbols such as a "smiley" (Table 2.7). These are made up of several characters typed in a row to form a larger figure. Smileys are an example of such "emoticons," icons for indicating emotions.

Mailing Lists

Mailing lists are an extension of e-mail used to send mail to the same group of people over an extended period. For example, a hospital could create an alias called "medical staff" that lists the e-mail addresses of all the staff physicians. To send a message to medical staff, they simply specify medical staff in the "To" line and the same message will be sent to everyone on that list (alias). Any

Table 2.7. Internet symbols for conveying emotion ("emoticons")

Emoticon (view sideways)	Meaning
:-)	Happy or smile
:-}	Ironic or wry smile
;-)	Wink
:-(or :-{	Sad or too bad
;-(or ;-{	Crying
<:-l	Dunce or hat
:+<	Hard night last night
:-o	Yawn or surprise
:-O	Shock
:o)	Friendly teddy bear
:-@	Screaming
:-Q	"Neener, neener" or smoking
:-p	Sticking out tongue
:*	Kiss or kissing
8-)	Glasses, shades, or amazement
::	Action markers, as in ::picks up gun and shoots computer::

incoming message sent to the mailing list "alias" is automatically sent to everyone on the mailing list. Some mailing lists are moderated or monitored by an electronic postmaster. This is especially common within organizations or companies. In these lists, a moderator reviews each incoming message for appropriateness and either passes it through for distribution or rejects it. Some moderators will also prepare *digests*, or a summary. The digest will contain a whole set of messages and articles in one package, making it much easier to keep up with a set of related information.

Mailing lists are maintained in two ways, either manually or by a specialized computer program. In the manual approach, the list administrator takes care of adding or deleting addresses from the master distribution list. In the program approach, you send messages to the address of a computer that provides this service. An example of this latter type is the mailing list maintained by the Centers for Disease Control, which electronically sends the contents of several of their publications to those who request them through an electronic message.

Legal Issues

Privacy, libel, and copyright are legal issues that impact e-mail users. Understand that privacy is *not* assured with electronic mail. There are no legal requirements that prevent an institution or company from reading incoming and outgoing e-mail messages. If you are using your employer's equipment, this is especially applicable. In addition, once you have sent a message, you have no control over what the recipient may do. He or she may send a copy to someone else without your knowledge. For the same reasons, do not assume that messages you receive are private. The sender may have sent the same message to others without using the "Copies to" function. If secure information must be sent, encryption programs such as PGP (Phil's Pretty Good Privacy, available at:

http://web.mit.edu/network/pgp.html) must be used. (The special issues of patient privacy will be discussed in Chapters 6 and 10.)

You should also be aware that even though you have deleted a mail message from your mailbox, you cannot assume that it has been completely erased. Many institutional and company policies require regular backups of their computer system disks, which generally hold incoming and outgoing mail messages. It is possible that a copy of your message was taken during a regular system backup. Be aware that your e-mail records can be subpoenaed, so care and periodic purging or clean up is advisable.

A second legal issue for e-mail users is libel. Libel is applicable within e-mail messages and newsgroups. Take care with your comments. What you say can be held against you.

Finally, copyright law applies to transferring files and information. It is illegal to distribute copyrighted information by any means, including electronic transfer. It is common to find material that has been scanned by a user for personal use and then distributed through e-mail. Unless the copyright owner has granted specific permission for the transfer of such material, it is illegal to do so.

Voice

Text is not the only form of data that may be sent over the Internet. Bi-directional transmission of voice (like a telephone) is now possible, thought it requires some minor hardware and software changes. To communicate this way, both the sending and receiving parties must be using the same protocols and software. A high-speed connection and computers with strong processing power are a must if the voice is to be lifelike and easily understood. For more information, software information, and downloads or technical specifications, check these sites:

> **http://www.telecoms-mag.com**
> **http://cws.internet.com/chat-ivc.html**
> **http://www.webattack.com/freeware/comm/fwvoice.shtml**
> **http://www.langner.com/english/products/luca_e/documentation/**
> **voice_transmission.html**

Video

Today's high-speed computers and Internet connections make it possible to send video data across the Internet in real time. (Though it won't look like a DVD just yet.) Video compression (using programs such as Apple's QuickTime) allows you to receive broadcasts of the BBC or CNN as streams of audio and video information. Teleconferencing is now possible on desktop machines, and there has been an explosion of "Webcams" that provide glimpses of everything from the passing of people in the street to game show contestants.

To receive most broadcasts of video information, simple browser plug-in programs are all that are required. It you want to be able to transmit or to carry out a videoconference, there are various kinds of equipment and software available. One combination that works well in the IBM/PC world is:

Microsoft Netmeeting 2.1 (a free software package)
Fast Internet connection—64kbps or faster (i.e.: ISDN, T-1, or cable modem on both sides)
Pentium 300 MHz or better
Any PCI based video capture card
Any NTSC video camera

Futher information about video transmission can be found at major computer manufacturer's Web sites or at

http://www.colorado.edu/CNS/Digit/septoct96/video.html

Security Issues

Much has been made of security and the Internet. We read news reports about hackers breaking into national defense computers, altering bank records, falsifying school records, and the like. Reports of computer viruses that can turn your computer into a toaster abound. There are strangers who entice your computer with "cookies." Paranoia over credit card number theft has made many shy away from Internet commerce. What is the reality? Like most things in life, there are risks, but the reality is that risks are small and can be easily reduced to acceptable levels. Let's take them one at a time.

Viruses

Viruses are small, free-running computer programs that are unwanted and perform functions that range from the irritating to the malicious. Somewhat like sexually transmitted diseases, these viruses are most often caught during indiscretions: exchanging software with strangers, getting something for nothing, or becoming intimate with strangers. Like sexual counterparts, they require the exchange of digital fluids (files). They are most likely to ride piggyback on floppy disks, but may be downloaded with files or e-mails from distant computers over the Internet. Programs from reputable software suppliers are low risk; shared files from a tacky bulletin board are not. Antivirus programs are readily available and are highly recommended. You can get more information on-line at **http://thunderbyte.com** (ThunderBYTE, Windows) or **http://charlotte.acns.nwu.edu/jln/progs.ssi** (John Noarstand's Disinfectant, Macintosh).

Most new computers come with some antivirus program installed. It is imperative that the user continuously updates the data set of the program so it can protect against new breeds of virus. Visiting the supplier's Web site easily does this. Some programs offer the ability to perform this update on an automatic basis. If this is an option with your software, take it; human nature suggests you won't do the update yourself until after you become infected.

Electronic mail cannot contain viruses; files attached to the message can. As a result, do not open attachments that you are not expecting or do not come from a trusted friend. If there is any doubt, check with the sender before opening the attachment. If you do not know the sender or there is any reason to be suspicious, through away the e-mail (and its attachment) without opening them. This will prevent the virus from being able to infect your machine or disks.

Cookies

Cookies are small files that are left on your computer, in the hard drive, by some Internet sites. These files are limited in size, can only be opened by the site that left them, and must contain an expiration date. They save information about you and your interaction with the distant computer's Web site. This information may contain when you last visited, your shirt size, type of computer you use, or your preference in books. The next time you visit that Web site, it can retrieve the cookie and use the information to customize its interaction with you. Yes, these do contain information that could be considered personal, but Web browser programs oversee the access and use of these files, limiting your risk. Most Web browsers allow you to be consulted before a cookie is "set." You can decide at that point whether to allow the cookie or not. If you are unsure and do not plan to visit the site often, you can "just say no."

Security and Credit Card Fraud

While it is possible to intercept data as it is being transmitted across the Internet in an effort to steal credit card numbers, the risk is very low. It is probably as risky or more so to give your credit card to the waiter in a restaurant. You should use the same care you would in other settings; if the establishment looks seedy and questionable, don't do it. The same holds for the Internet. Most Internet commerce sites will offer several options for payment including secure (encrypted) transmission of credit card information, C.O.D., or a 1-800 number to confirm your purchase.

Secure Transmissions

Most Internet browsers offer some forms of encryption option and many sites will invoke these options when they deal with sensitive of personal information. Examples range from on-line banking and credit card purchases, to viewing your frequent-flier mileage balance. Figure 2.6 illustrates the symbols displayed by both Netscape Navigator and Microsoft Internet Explorer.

Figure 2.6. Both Netscape Navigator (or Communicator) and Microsoft Internet Explorer indicate that an encrypted (secure) transaction is under way by placing an icon in the browser window. Shown are the icons from Netscape Communicator.

Encryption

Encryption takes the characters you enter and converts them into bits of code that are securely transmitted over the Internet. In other words, encryption is a process of using a key, also referred to as a cipher, to scramble readable text into text that can only be read by someone with the cipher for decrypting it. By doing this, even if the data that is transmitted is somehow intercepted, it cannot be read. This altered, meaningless data is what is referred to as ciphertext. Decryption changes the unreadable data back into its first form. There are various types of encryption such as private key encryption, public key encryption, digital signatures, and digital certificates. The full details of this rapidly growing field of mathematics and computer science are well beyond the scope of this book, but a good general review of the topic can be found at

http://www.utdallas.edu/~samit/ba4323/encrypt/encryption.html

Firewalls

A firewall is a system, including both hardware and software, that enforces access control between two networks. Specifically, a firewall is designed to allow someone to connect to the Internet, while preventing unauthorized users to gain access in the other direction. Usually network firewall software runs on a dedicated server connected to a hospital, university, or company's Intranet. The function of the server and its software is to examine incoming and outgoing packets and, according to a set of rules defined by the network administrator, either let them through or block them. Any computer that is continuously connected to the Internet should (ideally) be protected by a firewall. Good firewall programs are available for the individual user and should be considered if you use a cable modem, ISDN, or DSL connection that remains connected all of the time. Remember that firewalls do not provide virus protection. A separate type of software program must provide that protection.

When your computer is not connected to the Internet, the only way someone has access to your files and information is through your keyboard. When you connect to the Internet, your files are still closed to all but the most dedicated hackers, who have bigger fish to fry. If you have sensitive data, such as patient or financial information, some precautions are probably in order.

Internet Security Tips

Several simple steps will reduce the risk that your computer will be either the victim of an unwanted intrusion or the conduit by which other computers are entered:

- If you are connected to a network, do not attach a modem or other communication device to your computer without first discussing the proposed addition with your network administrator. This is one of the most common "backdoors" into a computer network and one of the easiest to avoid.

- If your computer is attached to a local network, turn it off when you are not using it. This not only saves power and prolongs the life of your monitor, but also makes it impossible to steal information if the machine is not running.
- Pick passwords that are not obvious. While you have to be able to remember your password, if it is readily apparent (your first name, your birth date, the digits of your Zip Code, local football mascot, or the name of your spouse), it is all too easy to make a guess and have open access. Consider using more esoteric information that is not available to others: your first grade teacher's name, the batting average of your sister, or the capital of Wyoming (no one ever remembers that). The best passwords are those that are a mixture of letters or letters and numbers that have no meaning. If your password system differentiates between cases, use mixed upper and lower case letters.
- Do not post your passwords or give them to anyone else, no matter how trusted. Passwords often become public in innocent ways without malicious intent. And yes, someone WILL find that sticky note you hid under the keyboard with your password written backwards on it.
- Change your password frequently. For high-security situations or files, consider changing it weekly; for most other situations a monthly change is sufficient. If necessary, use the first or last day of the month as a reminder. When you make this change, avoid choosing a new password that is related in an obvious way to the old password. Using sequences such as *password.1* followed by *password.2* and *password.3* is easier to remember, but defeats the purpose of making the change. Using sequences that make sense to you but would not be obvious to others may be acceptable.
- Many programs that deal with potentially sensitive material allow individual files to be password protected. If there is any doubt about security, or the contents of your files are sensitive, seriously consider using this option. This is true even at home if you do not want your kids looking through the checkbook program.
- If you have sensitive files and must remain connected to a network, consider placing these files on removable storage media. This might be a floppy disk, Zip disk, data cartridge, or similar device. The best hacker in the world can't get at files that are in you desk drawer.

Final Thoughts

If you connect to the Internet by telephone, you may want to consider a second telephone line. If you go this route, do not get fancy options like call waiting because they will knock you off your connection when they function. If you must have these options for other reasons, check with your local telephone company and ask them for the appropriate code to disable these features while a computer call is in progress.

Lastly, if you connect to the Internet when you travel, be very careful that you know the charges imposed by your hotel. Gone are the days of free local calls. Hotels see telephone connections to the Internet as both a threat and opportunity. They do not want to have all of their outgoing telephone lines tied up by daylong Internet connections, and telephone calls represent a lucrative profit center. Most hotels impose a fee for local calls, but increasingly they are moving to charges based on time, distance, or both. Consequently, although you may have verified that your Internet provider's telephone number is a local call, you may still be hit with a very large bill.

3
Finding the Information You Want

Almost anyone can become "connected." Once connected, anyone is free to place or retrieve information with no constraints on content, opinion, or quality. There are innumerable vetted sources of information and just as many of questionable value. Sites that catalog and search the information on the Internet make finding reliable sources that may be scattered anywhere around the globe easier. They are equally good at finding sites of less value or reliability. There are also some simple strategies that can make the process easier, more productive, and dependable.

Building a Strategy

If you view the process of finding information on the Internet as being analogous to tasks we perform daily, the process is less intimidating. As an example, suppose we wanted to buy a shirt. How would we go about it? We could rely on past experience and go to the place we got a shirt last time. We could ask someone where they bought their shirt. We could consult a directory, such as the phone book, or we could go to a place that sells many things (like a mall) and look for someone that sells shirts there. We could even employ a shopping service. Similar strategies will work to find information on the Internet.

Past Experience

If the information you are seeking is similar to that you have needed in the past, you may be able to use sites you have visited before, or the experience gained from those experiences, to help direct your search. If you are looking for specific content and you have seen the kind of thing you need at a site in the past, the chances are that you can get it again from the same location.

Web browsers incorporate a number of special features that make navigating on the Internet much more convenient. Two of the most powerful features are bookmarks (sometimes called "favorites") and search (or connection) histories. Bookmarks are a personal list of sites that the user wishes to keep for future reference. This list is maintained by the program and is available for use at any time the program is running (Fig. 3.1). These sites may be those that you need to visit frequently, or wish to return to later to explore more fully, or may represent a hard-to-find resource that may be required in the future. In addition to this list, the program also maintains a list of sites visited during the current session. This list is arranged in chronological order and is purged every time the program is exited. Using this connection history, it is easy for the user to explore a series of links and still return to an intermediate point from which to pursue yet another branch.

You can use experience to tell yourself what doesn't work. Suppose the last time you typed a technical term into your browser it didn't find the article you *knew* was in last year's journal. Your failure was probably because you were asking the wrong question of the wrong person (figuratively). You now know that if you want to get the contents of a journal article, you had better go to the Web site of that journal, to a specialty society, or, to a site with MedLine access. Those sites can help you while "www.technical_title.com" will not.

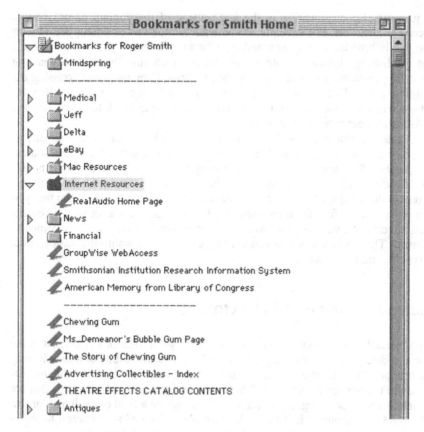

Figure 3.1. Bookmarks make returning to favorite sites much easier.

The Direct Approach

The simplest approach to get information over the Internet is to go directly to it. One option for this comes from the naming of Web sites by the Domain Name Service (DNS). Since humans do not remember the numerical addresses used internally by the Internet, sites are assigned unique names as placeholders. The person, corporation, or institution that operates the site chooses these names. The name chosen generally reflects the ownership of the site, content, or both. Consequently, **www.coke.com, www.toyota.com, and www.pbs.org** will take you to predictable locations. Because of this, if the information you seek is about a product or service, you may be able to directly type a word or phrase and link directly to the information you want.

Direct access will work best with certain types of information: General corporate or product information. Be aware that not every name will work. Cleaver web site owner have been known to use variants of popular names or to even second guess a company and register a brand or name before the obvious owner can. (New laws help protect against this type of abuse, but examples still exist.)

You must also be sensitive to the last portion of the domain name. This is ".com," ".org," etc. For example, if you want to look up something you saw on the public broadcasting system and type "**www.pbs.com**" you will get the site for Publishing Business Systems. To get the PBS (the Public Broadcasting System) you want, you will need "**www.pbs.org**." Even more embarrassing examples abound, including mistakes that will take you to adult sites (**www.whitehouse.com**). As a search strategy, this may work for some types of information, but most often it will not.

Another option is to use the site name provided by a product or company as a part of their advertising, product labeling, business letterhead, or other source. Corporate URLs now show up on everything from soup cans and magazine ads to the sides of city buses. If this is the information you seek, this is quick and direct. It does require that you have access to or remember the URL and that you are seeking the information the company is providing. Just as in print or broadcast advertising, you are somewhat at the company's mercy when it comes to content. This approach is best suited to times when you want information about a specific product or service.

Referrals (Portals and Directories)

Commercial and noncommercial sites offer listings of locations of interest in the form of directories or "link pages." These lists, like the results of a search, may be grouped for convenience and act as hypertext links that can take the user directly to the desired information. These lists will generally contain sites that are of interest to a specific group or interest. This may be a field of medicine, or site of interest to a group of hobbyists. An example of such a list of interest to medical professionals is one maintained by Slack Incorporated, located at

http://www.slackinc.com/areas.asp

This site offers a number of ways to access medically related information including its Medical Matrix listing (Fig. 3.2).

The use of lists maintained by commercial or organizational suppliers can often lead one directly to information when an appropriate search term is unknown. This is especially useful when the topic is one that is totally unfamiliar.

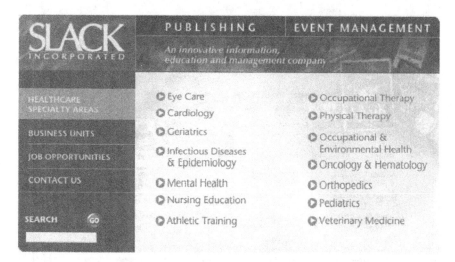

Figure 3.2. The site maintained by Slack Incorporated provides a list of Internet locations of interest to medical professionals, grouped by area of interest.

Shopping Services (Search Engines)

Web browsers have access to multiple search programs used to find Web sites that may contain information germane to the user's request. Services such as Yahoo, Magellan, Infoseek, and Lycos provide easy interfaces to the Web and its contents (Fig. 3.3). These search engines gather information about sites located on the Web by sending out "spiders" or "crawlers" that query each site they encounter and report back to the home computer on the contents they find. This information is classified and entered into a database or list that outside users can search. The utility of these databases is dependent on the frequency with which the scouts are sent out and the quality of the indexing that takes place in the database itself.

When using most of the search systems shown, a word or phrase is entered into the text block and the search button is clicked. Don't worry, advertisers, not the user, pay for the use of these search utilities. The program will return a series of possible links to other files or sites, often with a numerical index suggesting the degree of relevance to the search string. This index of relevance will give the user a sense of how likely a site is to contain the information sought. This helps to reduce time spent looking for information at a site that is semantically similar to the search term but unrelated to the desired content. The more specific the original search string is, the more likely it is that a limited number of relevant sites will be found, with few or no extraneous matches included. An example of such a search and its results are shown in Figure 3.4.

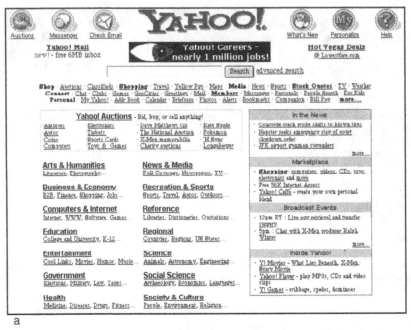

a

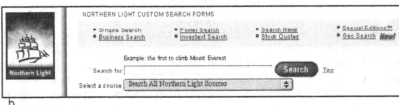

b

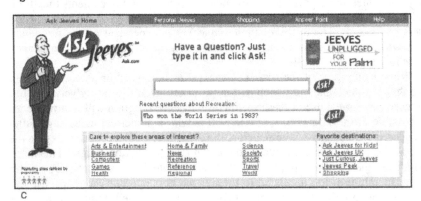

c

Figure 3.3. Web search engines provide powerful allies for finding information on the Internet. The interface used by these search engines is generally similar to those shown here for Yahoo (a), Northern Light (b), and Ask Jeeves (c). In many cases there are specific links to medical or health information that may be selected directly.

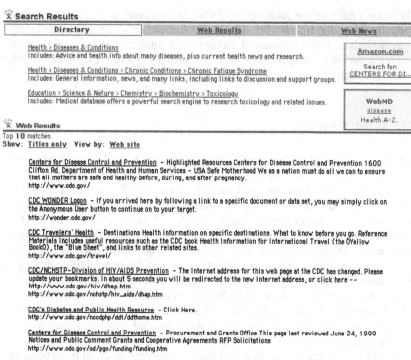

Figure 3.4. A typical search for "Centers for Disease Control" using the Excite search engine returns a number of possible sites. Some search engines will provide an indication of the degree to which they met the search criteria.

With most Web search engines, the results shown for any search are in the form of hypertext links that allow you to click on the desired entry and automatically connect with that site.

Search Agents

The concept of a search agent has become important in both Artificial Intelligence (AI) and mainstream computer science. Internet Search agents are software programs that reside on the user's computer, accept the information request (often in "natural language"), process the request using algorithms developed by artificial intelligence research, and then search the search engines. In short, they are search engines for search engines. (Technically, software agents differ from conventional software in that they are long-lived, semiautonomous, proactive, and adaptive, but for our purposes this definition will suffice.[2]) The advantage of these agents is their ability to synthesize the "intent" of the search and not just perform a verbatim query. The result for the user is increased ease of use (you don't have to know computer jargon or Boolean logic) and results that are more

---

[2] A good discussion of software agents can be found at the MIT media lab site: **http://belladonna.media.mit.edu/groups/agents/**

likely to be what you are looking for. There are versions of search agents that continually watch the Internet for information that fits criteria you supply. When the agent finds new information, it alerts you or automatically downloads the information for immediate display. We will further explore these "meta search engines" and their cousins, metabrowsers, below.

Start Your Engines

There are a number of Web search utilities from which to choose (Table 3.1). Given this richness, how should you choose the one to use? Although these services look similar, there are fundamental differences. Some, like Yahoo, are site directories that are lists, edited by humans, which are driven by topic. This type of search engine generally draws on a list of about 500,000 sites. That sounds like a lot until you realize that there are an estimated 100+ million pages of information on the Web (and growing daily). True search engines index the data contained on the Web pages themselves, not just the general topic that they cover. These engines use the spiders or crawlers mentioned above to retrieve detailed information from about 30 to 50 million pages of data. Consequently, if you are looking for a broad topic, a service such as Yahoo will give you the best results. If your needs are more specific or more detailed, search engines such as AltaVista or Excite will be of more help (Fig. 3.5). Some search engines, such as Google, offer "safe searching" that will filter the content to avoid objectionable sites. There are even "meta search engines" that combine the answers from several different engines (see below). Examples of this type are Dogpile and MetaCrawler. There is even one, NetShepherd, that offers filtering for "family-safe" content.

Table 3.1. Internet search utilities

Utility	Location (http://www.)
Ask Jeeves	ask.com
AltaVista	altavista.digital.com
Dogpile	dogpile.com
Excite	excite.com
HotBot	hotbot.com
Infoseek	infoseek.com
Lycos	lycos.cs.cmu.edu
MetaCrawler	metacrawler.com
NetShepherd	family.netshephard.com
Northern Light	northernlight.com
Webcrawler	webcrawler.com
Yahoo	yahoo.com

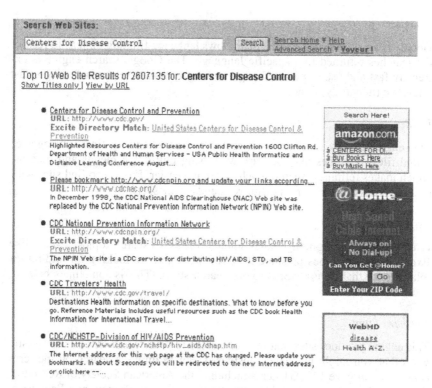

Figure 3.5. A typical search for "Centers for Disease Control" using the Excite search engine. Also visible is some of the advertising that pays for these services.

Let's review the five most commonly used search utilities:

Ask Jeeves

This engine is excellent for natural language general questions like how to tie a necktie or who won the World Series in 1937. As a general content search engine, this is not the most powerful resource for medical information, but useful for lots of other questions.

AltaVista

This engine is excellent for finely tuned, specific, or arcane references. The power of this search engine must be tempered with the use of Boolean logic commands such as AND or NOT to avoid being buried with unwanted sites. AltaVista wins as most powerful, but hard-to-master search engine.

Excite

Excite allows you to sort the results of large searches. This can be useful when your search returns more sites than there are HMO claims agents. This engine does not index links contained within Web pages and is often not intuitive about guessing what categories of information you are really after.

Google

Google is a newer search engine that allows language-filtering options to restrict the matches returned to a specific language. The Google search engine is extremely fast and uses a patented page ranking system to return sites of greatest relevance (hopefully) first.

HotBot

This engine is very good for more specific searches and for finding images or sound files. Searches may be narrowed using pull-down menus and buttons, which makes refining a search much faster and easier. It can also find sites with specific types of files such as pictures, sounds, games, etc.

Lycos

Excellent for finding images and sounds related to search topics, Lycos, like Excite, will sometimes presume it knows what you are looking for and return related sites that do not contain your search string. This is sometimes helpful, sometimes not.

Northern Light

This engine provides sites that may be related to your search criteria in heuristic ways that you might not have considered. For example, a search on the term *contraception* gave 121,031 items including the American Society of Reproductive Medicine, along with folders on the Pope and the Papacy, and Pediatrics. The ability to narrow your search and group items by relevance makes this an easy site to use.

Yahoo

As noted above, Yahoo is a topics-based searchable directory. While not the most powerful or comprehensive search utility, it is easy to use and well suited for day-to-day searching. It uses a plain-English search system and is good at matching what you may have meant in a nonspecific search.

Meta Search Engines and Metabrowsers

In the last several years there has been an emergence of programs that allow the user to search other search engines or customize the material they receive through the use of customized programs that replace their usual Internet browser. The simplest and most common of these are the meta search engines.

A meta search engine is nothing more than a program that interprets a user's search request, often entered as a common English sentence, and develops search strategies that are passed to other search engines. These may take the form of Internet-based sites such as Dogpile or MetaCrawler, or they may reside on the user's own computer such as MacIntosh's Sherlock search engine. Internet meta search sites tend to offer a dizzying set of options as they try to be a little of everything for everybody (Fig. 3.6). If your needs are for common sets of information such as stock quotes, travel information, and the like, these will be the fastest way to the specific information you need. They also offer direct links to sites that offer specific searchable information such as telephone directories, city guides, and government listings.

Another group of meta search engines are those that reside on your own computer, direct your search to other search sites, and then compile the results. A popular and particularly powerful one is MacIntosh's Sherlock. This program is used to search for file information on the user's computer or to retrieve information from the Internet. When used to search for Internet sites, a natural language request is entered (Fig. 3.7a) and the sites to be searched selected from a continuously updated list. The request is processed, sent to the selected sites, and possible matches returned. The results are sorted based on the program's assessment of relevance to your request and displayed (Fig. 3.7b). Information about the specific site can be displayed before the site is visited to help ensure the pertinence of the information.

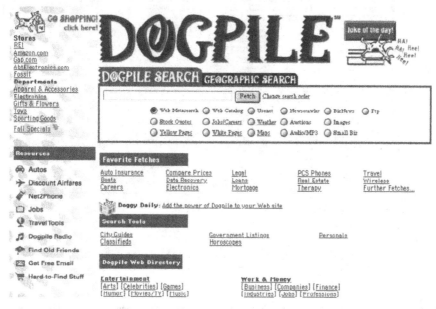

Figure 3.6. Dogpile.com is an example of a meta search site that offers precompiled searches and searches of other search engines. (**www.dogpile.com**)

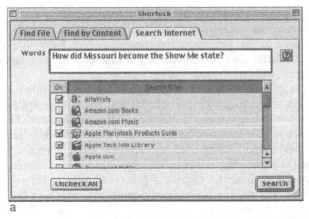

a

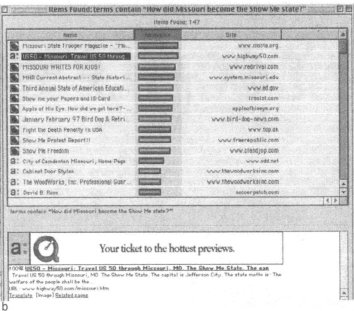

b

Figure 3.7. Sherlock, the MacIntosh's meta search program, accepts natural-language requests and searches other search engines as defined in a checklist (a). In this case, 147 responses ranked by estimated relevance were returned (b). Clicking on any listing gives more information in the box below.

Metabrowsers are designed to take the place of the usual Internet browser program and perform customizable functions not available in the standard system. Among the new tools, the most radical enable people to bypass the standard Web browser altogether by downloading graphic taskbars that are displayed directly on the computer desktop. Two examples of this type of services are Snippets and EntryPoint, which use a long, horizontal bar that sits at the bottom of your desktop screen. Another type is DoDots (for the Windows environment[3]), which features small square windows that hover on your desktop wherever you choose to put them. A Dot is a small package of Internet content delivered directly to your desktop. Choose what Dots you want and you can stay connected with information while working in other applications such as Word, Excel, or e-mail. For example, collect the TrafficStation Dot and you can check the traffic at any time without going to the Web site, the weather dot will keep you appraised of the weather, and so on. Other programs work within the format of the standard Web browser but tweak it. Programs such as those from Neo-Planet or InfoGate offer the chance to alter the Internet Explorer browsers with colors and patterns while adding buttons for their favorite sites, weather reports, and news headlines. Another service, HotBar.com, offers similar options for both Netscape and Internet Explorer browsers. The developers of both Internet Explorer and Netscape are unveiling new browsing tools that have similar capabilities. Netscape 6, which has just been introduced, includes tabs on the left side of the browser that can be customized to include pieces of Web content. Microsoft's latest version of Internet Explorer, 5.5, allows you to create buttons that link to frequently used Web sites.

While these customized browsers are not search engines, and vice versa, these new meta browsers and customized information delivery systems are designed to reduce the user's dependence on traditional search engines. They also strive to ensure that the searches that are performed return a greater percentage of useful sites. In the short term, however, the drawbacks of the services could outweigh their benefits. To get these features, for example, users will often have to divulge details about themselves such as zip code, stock holdings, or new preferences. Snippets asks for the user's sex, zip code, job interests, and e-mail address. DoDots collects data about how often a user turns to its services, how long is spent with the services, and what information is sought. In both cases, the companies tell their customers how they use the data, and many people may be willing to sacrifice some privacy for convenience. Despite these promises, privacy is not completely assured. A recent example is that of Amazon.com, in which the company changed course in midstream and decided to distribute its customers' personal data if they bought products from other vendors at the Amazon site. The stand-alone programs like DoDots or Snippets have essentially opened a new gateway for information to travel into and out of your computer. Just as we pointed out the need for a firewall if you remain continuously connected to the Internet, these programs open a channel through which information may pass without your knowledge.

With any new software that you install, there is the possibility of conflicts with existing software of operating systems—a notorious problem in the Windows operating environment. Another concern to be aware of is that any program that is designed to run continuously (as these are) may be difficult to get rid of if you should have problems or tire of its function. Metabrowsers represent an efficient way to access Internet information, but for the moment they will not replace the traditional methods of access and searching.

---

[3] Requires Windows 95, 98, 2000 and NT4. Supports Internet Explorer 4+, Netscape 4.72+, & AOL 5+.

General Search Secrets

Effective searches, that is, ones that don't waste time and give you sites that fit your needs, are relatively easy if you follow some simple suggestions:

- In many search engines, if you capitalize a word of text in your search request, only words matching that capitalization will be matched; lower case words will match independent of case. Therefore, use capitals (and accent characters as well) only when necessary.
- Place double quotes (" ") around words that should be treated as a single phrase. Without the quotes the search engine may return sites that contain the words, but separated by pages of other text.
- In many search engines you can place a plus sign (+) or a minus sign (–) in front of words that must or must not be a part of the documents found. (If used, there must be a space before the sign and not between the sign and the specific word. If in doubt, check to see if your search engine offers search tips or an "advanced" mode to help give you specifics for that engine.)
- Be aware, many search engines will ignore punctuation and treat the elements as if they were separate search parameters. This results in U.S.A. returning anything with an upper-case A, an upper-case S, or an upper-case U, which is not the same as a search for USA.
- Many search engines have the ability to use logical statements such as AND, OR, and NOT, but these may only be available in the "advanced" mode. Check the specific search engine for details.
- If you are unsure, start with the most general search terms and then refine the search based on the initial results. When you are sure, use the reverse strategy—start with the most specific search terms, and broaden the search as needed.
- Most search engines allow "wild card" characters such as * in the search string. These characters allow one or more characters to match. For example, the search for ultraso* would match ultrasonography or ultrasound. (Be careful, it might also give you ultrasophisticated.)
- Try to be specific when you can. Searching for a phrase like "ultrasonography breast cyst benign" is better than "breast" or "breast disease." (We will deal with the pornography issue later.)
- If you find something useful, consider bookmarking it or saving it on your computer's hard disk.

Remember that these search techniques find the location of Web sites. If you are looking for specific content, such as a journal article, you should be looking within a site, not at the site itself. Think before you search. No Web browser will find the information available to a MedLine search, and MedLine cannot tell you about Web sites.

4
Becoming a Presence on the Internet

Many times, the decision to become a part of the Internet goes beyond the usual surfing to actually developing a presence on the Web. This varies from the posting of a home page for family and friends so they can keep up on news, photographs, or a hobby, to developing an informational or interactive site dealing with a medical issue or practice development. Many Internet service providers make space available on their computers for such Web sites, and the languages used to compose and display a Web page are easily mastered. In this chapter we explore the basics of putting up a Web page. While all the nuances of Web programming are beyond the scope of this book, this chapter should allow you to put up a respectable-looking page and get you started as a Webmaster.

What Is a Web Page?

A Web page is a text file containing instructions that tell a Web browser what information you would like displayed and how to display it. This display may contain family, business, hobby, political, or other content. The text file is written in HTML (HyperText Markup Language) or one of its enhancements and will contain pointers or "links" to other files or Internet sites. If you want the world to see your Web page, the Web page file or files must reside on a computer connected to the Web. Many value-added providers and regular Internet service providers make a limited amount of space available for this purpose as a part of their service. An example of such a hosting service is GeoCites (**http://www.geocities.com**), which offers free Web page hosting for non-commercial use.

Many organizations use Web pages located on internal networks that are shielded from the rest of the Internet by software or hardware blockades called firewalls. These Web pages are created in much the same way; they just play to a smaller audience.

Why Have a Web Page?

There are many reasons to have a "home page." You may want to keep friends and family current about your activities, let them see your new dog, or review prenatal ultrasounds (see security and the Interent, below). You might want to advertise your practice, or provide information for patients. This might take the form of frequently asked questions, office policies, or information about medical news of interest to your patients. You might like to publish your ideas or creations, promote a hobby, or help a charitable organization. There are almost as many reasons as there are Web pages.

Web Site Construction

Web pages are text written in HTML or its descendants. HTML consists of a series of commands or "tags" that tell the browser program how to handle the information you supply. This series of commands may be entered directly in your Web browser or word processing program by modifying samples or by using an HTML editing program. Editing programs make it fast and as easy to create Web pages as it is to create printed materials in a word processing program. The editor automatically places the appropriate tags in a text document to describe the function of the various parts of the text, such as addresses, headings, lists, quotes, and words to be emphasized. The HTML language is not that difficult, so direct entry for simple pages is a practical option as well. The final file of instructions is usually stored with the extension .html or .htm.

The HTML language allows you to use references to items, rather than the item itself. This saves programming time and space within your HTML file. Let's assume you wanted a picture of the front of your hospital or office to appear on each page of text you display. You could either include a copy of it on each page or simply insert a reference to where the picture is stored and allow the browser to insert it when needed. Now you get the idea. This flexibility also allows each browser to modify the look of the page based on screen size, resolution, number of colors that can be displayed, and other factors. While this loss of direct control seems like a throwback from the ability to control the look of the page directly—what you see is what you get (WYSWYG)—the fact that different browsers on different machines and monitors will have to interpret the information demands this type of display flexibility.

HTML Codes

HTML tags are code names surrounded by an open and closed angle bracket (<, >). Most tags require pairs of commands to turn functions on and off. Examples of this using the hypothetical command <BOLD> are these lines:

<BOLD>This line will be displayed in bold</BOLD>
In this line, only the word<BOLD>bold</BOLD> is highlighted

When displayed by the browser these lines will look like this:

This line will be displayed in bold
In this line, only the word **bold** is highlighted

When paired commands are used, the closing tag is preceded by a slash (/) telling the browser to turn off that command at that point. When the browser program reads the HTML page, it will format tagged text for display. Some examples of common HTML tags are shown in Table 4.1. Many additional commands are available to further change the look of your page.

Table 4.1. Common HTML tags

Tag	Meaning
<A>...</A>	Hypertext link
<ADDRESS>... </ADDRESS>	Displays enclosed text in address style
<BLOCKQUOTE>... </BLOCKQUOTE>	Displays text as indented block of text; often used for text quoted from another source
 	Starts a new line within a paragraph
<DIV ALIGN="???">... </DIV>	Aligns text based on *???* (right, left, or center)
<Hn>...</Hn>	Heading level n, from H1 (largest) to H6 (smallest)
<HR>	Horizontal line
<LI>	Item in a list
<OL>...</OL>	Ordered list (generally numbered items)
<UL>...</UL>	Unordered list (generally bulleted)
<P>	New paragraph (with blank line)
<PRE>...</PRE>	Preformatted text to be displayed as is
<EM...</EM>	Emphasizes enclosed text (usually underlined)
<STRONG>... </STRONG>	Displays text in bold (or strong emphasis style)
<I>...</I>	Displays text in italics
<B>...</B>	Displays text in bold
<TT>...</TT>	Displays text in monospace (typewriter) text
<META>...</META>	Information used by indexing programs and not for display
<TABLE>... </TABLE>	Defines the start and end of table style information (best used only with an editor)

All Web pages have the same basic elements:

<HTML><HEAD><TITLE>*Title text, not displayed*</TITLE></HEAD>
<BODY>
Material that makes up the body of the page
</BODY>
</HTML>

Because browsers will ignore extra spaces, tabs, and returns, these standard elements may be arranged for ease of viewing. The <HTML> and </HTML> tags identify the enclosed contents as HTML code. As more versions of markup languages appear, these become more important. The <HEAD> and </HEAD> tags indicate material that is not for display but is used by indexing programs to help users find your pages. The title included in the <HEAD> material is used for both indexing and as the label displayed by the bookmark feature of most browsers. Tags must also enclose the body of material that makes up the content of your page. Comments to make future editing easier may be added using the <COMMENT>…</COMMENT> tags.

You can experiment with this simplest form of Web page by typing in the above structure (inserting your own information for the italicized placeholders) in your favorite word processing program. Save the file with a simple (eight character IBM style) name and the ".htm" file type. You can then view your handiwork by starting your browser program and choose "OPEN" from its menu. Specify your file and step back to admire your work.

The font displayed on your page can be modified using the command:

<FONT FACE=*Times New Roman* SIZE=5 COLOR="*olive*">*text*</FONT>

The size of the display may be varied from 1 (very small) to 7 (very large) with 3 as the default setting. Allowable colors are white, black, red, green, blue, yellow, aqua, fuchsia, gray, lime, maroon, purple, navy, olive, silver, and teal. Typefaces allowed are based on what is installed on the system being used. Because you can't be sure about the fonts the viewing computer may have, it is best to stay with the old favorites. Mixing of lots of fonts, colors, and sizes is very distracting. Once again, less is more.

Pointers to other Web pages (one of the most useful aspects of Web browsers and HTML) are added with the following tags:

<A HREF=*Web URL*>*Text label to be displayed*</A>

In use this is how it might look:

<A HREF=http://www.umkc.edu>The Truman Medical Center</A>

The same format can be used to help users navigate within your own Web page by labeling a destination with a name using

<A NAME=*Label*></A>

The location is then called using the tag

<A HREF="#*Label*>*text prompt*</A>

This type of internal link is used to perform tasks such as skipping to start or end of long text passages, jumping to a specific topic, or returning to your starting point.

Images are just as easy to include in your page using the tag

<div align="center"><IMG SRC=“<em>picturename</em>”></div>

This tag is placed where you want the image displayed. The file must be located in the same computer folder as the HTML file for this command to work as shown. Generally a text string is added as an alternative (ALT=“text”) so that if the file is not found or cannot be displayed, the user will have some idea of what you intended. In a similar manner, the alignment of the image may be specified with the ALIGN tag, though when combined with other commands the “DIV” is omitted. When the image to point to is located on another source (host, folder, or computer), the HREF tag may be used as follows:

<div align="center"><A HREF=<em>URL</em>><IMG SRC=“<em>picturename</em>” ALIGN=“center” ALT
=“<em>text label</em>”></div>

Several HTML editors are available and are worth the investment if you are going to do much Web site creation or editing. Editors are included in the current versions of Netscape Communicator (4.7) or current Windows systems (called FrontPage Express). Microsoft Word and WordPerfect also offer the ability to edit Web pages. Shareware editors are available on line from

BBEdit Lite (Macintosh): http://www.barebones.com
Hot Dog Web Editor (Windows): http://www.sausage.com

Several extensions to the HTML language are available but beyond the scope of this book. They make it possible to have images with “hot spots” that can be clicked to send the user to a link, have sections of the screen (frames) that act as independently controlled sections, or contain forms where the user can fill in data. Moving and three-dimensional images may also be added in these dynamic HTML, XML, and VRML versions of the basic HTML language.

Once you are happy with the content and look of your Web page, it must be uploaded to the Web server that will act as host for your site. Instructions for this process are available from your Internet provider or Web server. Once your site is loaded, you should check it directly from the Web to ensure it is working as expected now that it is on the server. That's all there is to it: You are now “on the Web.”

Tips for Effective Web Pages

For the best Web pages, the following guidelines are recommended:

- Spend time surfing before you start to develop your own pages. All Web browsers have an option to directly view the HTML source code for the page you are viewing. When you find something you like, look at how the author accomplished the look or function. Most browsers allow you to save a copy of the HTML code on your hard disk so you can edit it in your word processor program and see the effects of your changes.

- Know what you want to accomplish with your Web page. The more clear your focus, the better the Web site.
- Be sure that your Web page(s) will be hosted on a reliable server with sufficient power to supply stable service in times of heavy traffic.
- Content (like neatness) counts. Nobody is interested in a site that is "just there." Provide content in the form of text, images, and useful and well-maintained links to other pages. Don't forget to check your spelling!
- Provide something to draw the visitor in at the very start of the Web page. Tell them what your page is about, and why they will want to visit. Pique their curiosity. Many casual visitors will stay only a few seconds if you do not grab their attention.
- Keep it simple. Just as with the warning about text made above, too many frills, fancy colors or backgrounds, spinning wheels, or animated logos distract and slow down the loading of the page. Most surfers won't wait to figure it all out. Keeping it simple also reduces the problems induced by different browsers, screen sizes, modem speeds, etc.
- Provide key words in the first paragraph or two for indexing purposes. You should also make liberal use of the <META> command to provide your own index terms.
- If you have more than one page; provide a link back to your main page.
- DO NOT include copyrighted material without permission. This includes images and text. If you are not sure material is in the public domain, don't use it. If you use an organization's name or persona, be sure you are authorized to speak for that group. Even if it is for your practice group, make sure the other members know what you are doing. This is one time when permission is preferable to forgiveness.
- Maintain any link you provide. Check it periodically to be sure that it is still on the Web and still has the content you expect. A link that leads to blind alley, or worse, reflects badly on you and your site.
- Periodically test your Web page to be sure it is working as you expect. Changes and updates to the browser can occasionally make a difference in how your page will look or function in the new version.
- Consider including your e-mail address and invite comments. This can be helpful if you are trying to promote your practice or encourage the exchange of information.
- Limit the amount of personal information you include. Not only are most of us not really interested, there are some risks. Putting in information about a recent gymnastic award displays your pride but could provide a plausible excuse for a stranger to take your child from school in the middle of the day.

- If you collect information from Web site visitors, provide a clear statement of your policies regarding the use and privacy of this information.

Security and the Internet

A great deal has been said about the Internet and hackers (those who, for sport or otherwise, break into computers connected to the Internet; crackers are those who do it for malicious purposes). It is true that if you are connected to the Internet, your computer may be vulnerable to access by someone else. Once hackers have access to your computer, they have access to all of the information stored on attached hard disks and to the information stored on any other computer connected to your computer by a local network. There are a number of software programs designed to limit access (called firewalls), but the persistent and dedicated hacker can circumvent even these. For casual users, like most physicians, the risks are minimal; we are generally only temporarily and sporadically connected to the Internet, and even then it is most often indirectly through the auspices of an Internet Service Provider (ISP). If you are going to be a serious presence on the Web, rather than a casual user, you should consider using a Web server that is not attached to the rest of your network, or securing the advice of a computer consultant regarding firewalls and other protective measures.

5
Patient Education and Information

Just as physicians are using the Internet to find current medical information, patients are doing the same thing—and they are doing it on a daily basis. Direct-to-consumer advertising by drug makers and Webmasters urge our patients to check out their Web sites. Patients call for information about the suitability of a particular prescription medication before a pharmaceutical sales representative has visited their physician. Patients frequently come for appointments armed with printouts of information obtained through the Internet. The ability of patients to access directly the same information that is available to their physician is a powerful example of the concept of disintermediation introduced in Chapter 1. Sometimes this ability is helpful, with information that is accurate and complete; sometimes it is dangerously out of date, inaccurate, or just plain wrong.

Computers and Patient Education

Point-of-service computer technology is used for patient education in two broad ways. The first method uses a computer to generate all the text and graphics displayed on the computer screen. This approach is limited by the substantial amount of keyboard interaction between the patient and the computer that was usually required. Several commercial programs of this type, including some that circumvent the keyboard with touch screens or light pens, are available for use in both office and hospital settings.

A second and much more powerful approach to computer-aided patient instruction is to use a computer in conjunction with another device. Examples of this are the combinations of a computer with a videotape, videodisk, or

CD-ROM (DVD) system. (An expanded collection of multimedia files on a high-speed hard disk system can perform the same function.) This system provides the visual quality of the original presentations and allows existing films and videotapes to be easily incorporated into the interaction. Patients can select a topic by choosing an option from a list that appears on the video screen. They can then use the computer to control both the speed and the progress of the educational process. This is somewhat analogous to the scene selection capabilities provided by standard DVD players, but the scene may be chosen by either the user or the computer software managing the interaction. This simplicity of operation, along with the high quality of the visual presentations, makes the combined video-computer combination a logical choice. Cost and the availability of materials of appropriate content and verification for a given practice setting have severely limited this approach, though some notable examples still exist.

The Patient Education Institute, located at the University of Iowa's Technology Innovation Center, provides software to help patients make educated health-related decisions and take an active role in their health care. The institue offers a software system titled X-Plain. X-Plain can be delivered on CD-ROM to run on existing computers, on X-Plain touch-screen kiosks, or over the Internet. The X-Plain software presents information using text, illustrations, animations, and narration. X-Plain also asks questions, gives responses, prints handouts, and documents education. Modules are currently offered in 15 different areas with more under development. The system only runs on the IBM (or IBM clone) platform. The single-user licensing fee is currently $495 per X-Plain module. The Patient Education Institute's Internet page (**http://www.patient-education.com/**) also contains links to the University of Iowa's Virtual Hospital patient education site (**http://www.vh.org/Patients/**), which contains patient education materials arranged by topic and specialty of the author (Fig. 5.1). The site also has links to educational materials for health care providers in the form of multimedia textbooks, teaching files, patient simulations, and lectures.

Bridging the gap between desktop-based in-office systems and those that are fully Internet based are some hybrid commercial sites that offer aspects of both systems to fill the need for educational systems. Examples include Medifor Direct (**http://www.medifor.com**) (Fig. 5.2), MediVation's provider-patient interface (**http://www.MediVation.com**), and Salu.net (**http://www.Salu.net**). These services work in conjunction with patient information provided by the physician or office staff. Each system offers secure access to patient information regarding medications, diagnosis, and other relevant information. This information may be either provided by the practitioner or obtained directly from an associated practice management package. In some instances, the service is free (Salu.net, Fig. 5.3), and in others subscriptions or fees are required for the use of the service. For the most part, services such as these are designed to provide their interaction within the office setting and are not directly accessible by the patients themselves. This allows for customization of the information provided, but requires more interaction and involvement by the physician or the office staff.

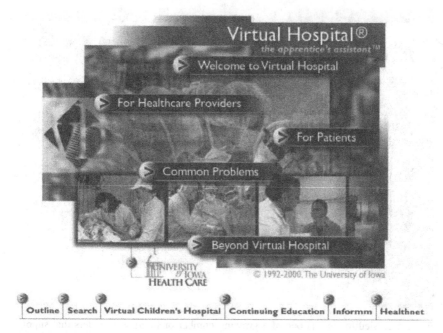

Figure 5.1. The University of Iowa maintains the Virtual Hospital site for patient education. (**http://www.vh.org**)

A different approach to patient education is the Internet based U-Write.com. This site offers to help create printed patient education materials for use within a practice (**http://www.u-write.com**). While it could be argued that this is not truly Internet patient education, the exchange of information and services that this site entails make it a part of the patient education resources available on the Internet.

In contrast to the paucity of computer education systems for the clinical setting, patient education or patient-accessible Internet sites abound. From support groups to public pages by major medical organizations, health care information on the Web has expanded rapidly. Just as in other arenas, the quality of the information available on the Internet is dependent on the individual or organization that posts the pages. Consequently, many practices choose to screen relevant sites and prepare lists of vetted sites with appropriate content. These lists may be provided to patients in print form or as links located on the practice's Web site.

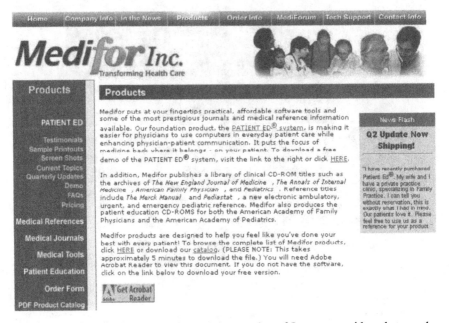

Figure 5.2. Medifor Inc. is one of a growing number of Internet providers that supply patient customized education and care instructions. (**http://www.medifor.com**)

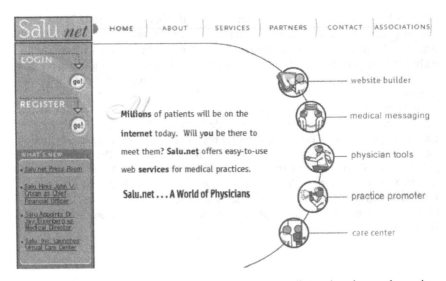

Figure 5.3. Salu.net provides a number of patient counseling, education, and practice promotion tools through its Web site. (**http://www.Salu.net**)

What Your Patients Are Seeing

Where medical information was once the exclusive province of health care providers to be dispensed on a one-to-one basis, now anyone with an Internet connection can perform medical literature searches, query professional associations, or join a support group. Our patients now have as much or more information at their fingertips as we do, and they have more time to find it than we do. This means that we must have some sense of the information and resources our patients have available.

General Sites

There ia a large and growing number of consumer-oriented medical information sites accessible via the Internet. Some are high profile, advertising directly to consumers through broadcast and print advertising; others are lower profile but equally accessible. An example of a widely advertised consumer site is Healtheon/WebMD (**http://www.webmd.com/**, Fig. 5.4). This site contains health information and services aimed primarily at consumers. In a nod to professionals, the site also offers a "physician" side that requires registration and a monthly fee. (At the time of this writing the fee is $29.95 per month, but a grant pays this fee for the first year, after which you are given the opportunity to continue at your own expense or discontinue your membership.) This fee entitles you to access the electronic version of Scientific American Medicine, news, and continuing medical education offerings. The site also offers billing assistance and purchasing information that is targeted to medical office managers.

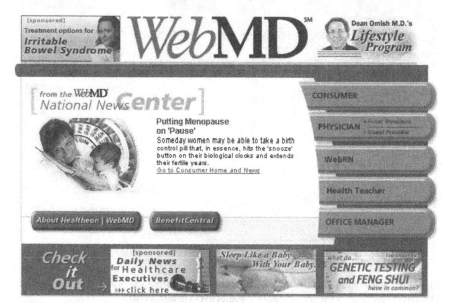

Figure 5.4. Healtheon/WebMD offers a variety of consumer-targeted health information and services. (**http://www.webmd.com/**)

The direct to consumer health market has prompted a number of diverse corporations to become involved with Web-based health information services. An example is the Discovery television channel's consumer health service, Discovery Health (**http://www.discoveryhealth.com**, Fig. 5.5). Like many other consumer health pages, the cost of this service is paid for by advertisers who buy space for banners, links, and other messages. (Many similar sites also offer product sales or electronic shopping, which helps to pay costs.) Like most other consumer sites, this site offers news stories, discussion of health topics, and disease specific information ranging from allergies to weight management. The information is grouped by general interest areas and by diseases or conditions. The site's information can be searched with a simple search engine that returns both the specific item requested and information that may (or may not) be relevant or of interest (although a try using the search term "contraception" led to a blank page). The material is a mixture of text and information written for the site or supplied from other sources. In some cases, the text is the transcript of lectures given at various conferences. As such, the style, depth, and content vary significantly. The source is annotated so that its reliability can be judged, but this is often difficult for someone who is not familiar with the field, the speaker, or the meeting where the information was presented.

Another example of a commercial site (and the hyperbole that often accompanies these efforts) is that offered by the successor of NetMed, MDChoice.com (**http://www.mdchoice.com**, Fig. 5.6). This site claims to be "the

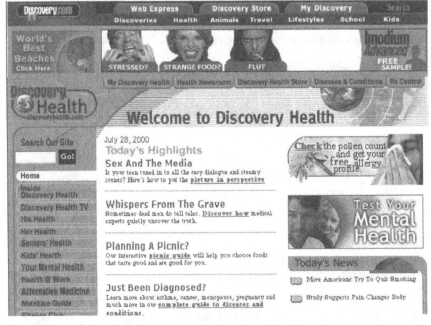

Figure 5.5. Discovery Health is the consumer health information portal provided by the Discovery television channel. (**http://www.discoveryhealth.com**)

ultimate medical information finder" and offers news, patient information grouped by topic, a search engine for the site, links to Medline, and other services. Interestingly, the Medline link is provided on the patient side of the site, but not on the physician's side. On the professional site, a search engine offers to provide articles that have been "selected by board-certified physicians," a feature that may or may not be advantageous, since we do not know the who and how of this process. This side of the site is not restricted and there is no fee for access, allowing patients and practitioners equal access. A link to a cardiac resuscitation simulator that may be of interest to professionals is provided, but potentially confusing to patients who happen to wander in by mistake.

A collaboration of Harvard Medical School and InteliHealth has led to the creation the InteliHealth consumer site (**http://www.intelihealth.com**, Fig. 5.7). This site provides the somewhat standard access to disease-specific information and news stories along with a commercial store for health-related products and services. This site offers the chance to sign up to receive free e-mails on specific medical topics from AIDS to women's health and 15 others in between. The interface at this site is more cluttered than some and does not display well if your browser is set to a narrow size or your screen resolution is not up to standard. The Harvard name provides some level of perceived authority that is missing from other completely commercial sites. As with many health-related sites, a certain level of prior medical knowledge and sophistication is helpful to

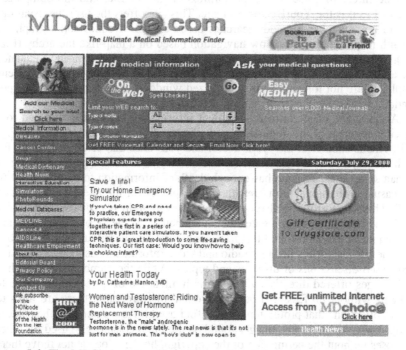

Figure 5.6. The MDChoice site offers news, patient information grouped by topic, a search engine for the site, links to Medline, and other services. (**http://www.mdchoice. com**)

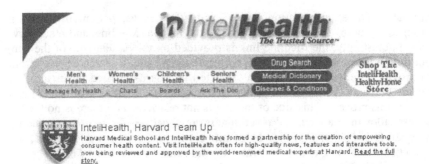

Figure 5.7. The InteliHealth site has content produced in collaboration with Harvard Medical School. (**http://www.intelihealth.com**)

get the most information. This aspect of all patient information sites potentially limits their utility for the medically naive.

One interesting use of the capabilities of the Internet and the computers attached to it is the YourDoctor.com site. This site offers the user the usual option of text searches but adds searches based on ICD-9 codes and a graphical "health map" interface to allow navigation based on a map-like hierarchy (Fig. 5.8). This interface is clearly different but requires a special plug-in to enhance the abilities of both the Netscape and Internet Explorer browsers. The screens displayed are not tolerant of different sized windows or screen resolutions, potentially weakening their appeal if the settings are not correct.

An example of a commercial patient information site that is targeted to a specific segment of the population is medispecialty.com's site, obgyn.net (Fig. 5.9). This is another of the "your doctor and you" sites that offers something for both the patient and the provider, but this one seems to make a better showing of it than some sites. The site has enough depth of information to be of interest to the casual professional with breadth and simplicity for the interested patient as well. This same group is also developing sites to address pediatric and family medicine issues. When you enter the area labeled "women's pavilion," you are offered news, resources, and features along with the ubiquitous search capability. The site also offers images, audio and video information, as well as the usual text-based discussions of diseases and topics. While the number of audio clips and images offered directly by the site is limited and of questionable value to patients without professional perspective and interpretation, there are links to other collections that professionals may find useful. As we note in other places in this book, be aware that images found on the Internet cannot be used for other purposes without the permission of the copyright holder. You cannot move them into a slide presentation or put them on your own Web site without permission. When in doubt, ask.

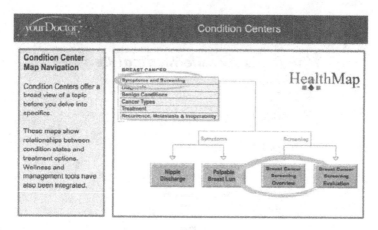

Figure 5.8. The site YourDoctor.com uses a graphical hierarchy for users to navigate when finding information. (**http://www.yourdoctor.com**)

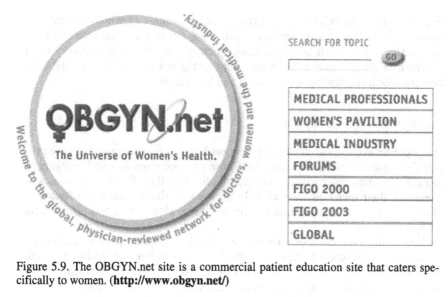

Figure 5.9. The OBGYN.net site is a commercial patient education site that caters specifically to women. (**http://www.obgyn.net/**)

Not all patient education sites are commercial or have commercial interest. Some sites are private or the altruistic work of charitable or other public agencies. An international example of a private site is one by Whitfors Avenue Medical Center in Perth Australia (Fig. 5.10). Some of the links provided point users back to sites in the United States, such as the virtual hospital mentioned above. This site points out one of the problems of Internet-based patient education; if patients are not Web-savvy or paying attention, they may never notice that they are looking at a site outside of their home country. With an offshore information provider, the information supplied may be appropriate for,

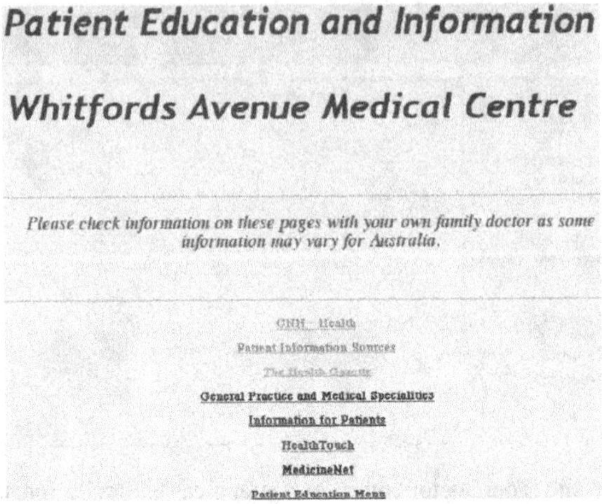

Patient Education and Information

Whitfords Avenue Medical Centre

Please check information on these pages with your own family doctor as some information may vary for Australia.

GNH   Health

Patient Information Sources

The Health Gazette

General Practice and Medical Specialties

Information for Patients

HealthTouch

MedicineNet

Patient Education Menu

Figure 5.10. This portal to patient information is maintained by a private medical clinic in Perth, Australia. (**http://members.iinet.net.au/~whitford/patient.html**)

or governed by, different rules or expectations than those to which the surfer is accustomed. In this case, a warning is provided, but in many instances no such informational warning is supplied. Consequently, patients could find very valid information about a new drug or treatment that is not approved or available in their own location, leading to confusion and frustration.

Organizations

Many public agencies as well as professional and charitable organizations provide patient information Internet sites. These sites are often less wide ranging in content than their commercial counterparts, limiting their focus to the topics of interest to their own constituencies. In most cases, these areas are sufficiently broad and apparent that Internet surfers should be able to find and utilize them easily.

 One of the most obvious sources for publicly supported patient (and other) information is the site maintained by the National Institutes of Health. Through this portal (Fig. 5.11) patients (and providers) can obtain news and information, and links to scientific and grant resources, and can connect to MedLine. Consumers can access a wealth of information about clinical trials, publications, and hot lines. Information is available about special programs and initiatives including rare diseases and the role of minorities in health research. The site is well organized, with both the depth and breadth you would expect from a government site, but it also has a surprisingly light touch that should make patients more comfortable. An example of this is the page that allows the user to search for disease- or condition-specific information—the NIH Health Information Index (Fig. 5.12). This index connects the user to the appropriate National Institutes section or government agency where more information can be obtained. Unlike some government programs, this page is easy to use, intuitive, functional, and lacking in stuffiness.

Many other government agencies offer access to patient information materials and can be useful for patients and providers alike (Fig. 5.13). Most government sites are easy to locate and can be identified by the ".gov" suffix. You can also us the new government site compilation at **www.searchgov.com**. This site provides links to most state and federal Web sites. The site also connects to independent agencies such as Amtrak and the Postal Rate Commission. If you do not use the search engine provided, it is helpful to know all the arcane abbreviations used by these agencies.

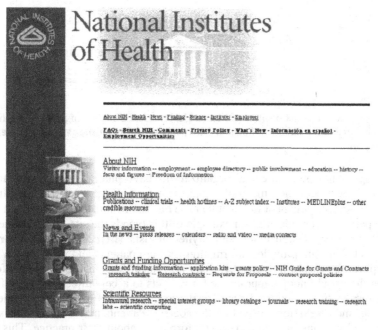

Figure 5.11. The National Institutes of Health offer electronic information for patients and practitioners through their Web site. (**http://www.nih.gov**)

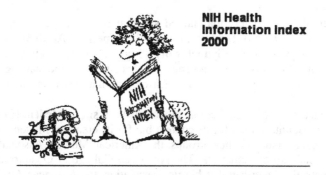

Figure 5.12. With a style and humor not usually associated with a government site, the NIH Health Information Index is a useful portal to patient information. (**http:// www.nih.gov/health**)

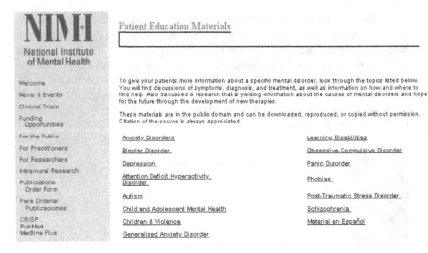

Figure 5.13. The National Institute of Mental Health offers a number of patient education materials, including many in Spanish. (**http://www.nimh.nih.gov/practitioners/patinfo.cfm**)

Many, if not most, medical organizations have public Internet sites that provide patient education materials along with password protected information and services for organization members. This is the most common form of vetted patient-accessible site. An example of this type is the site for The American College of Obstetricians and Gynecologists (**http://www.acog.org**, Fig. 5.14). This site provides information for both patients and members. With an appropriate password, members can access professional and other information that would not be appropriate for patients to access directly without further interpretation or counseling. Patients do have access to published patient materials and discussions hosted by the society. Patients may also use this site to locate physicians by area and view information about their practice. This referral capability is becoming more common and can be a useful method of practice promotion. (For more on using the Internet for practice promotion, see Chapter 10.)

An example of a society-maintained site that is separate from the site for member use is the Family Doctor site from the American Academy of Family Physicians (**http://www.familydoctor.org**, Fig. 5.15). A mixture of health tips, news, and disease-specific information, this site is a good starting point to refer patients to who want general information that has been screened for accuracy.

An unusual form of organization-supported Web site is Medem (Fig. 5.16). This site is most unusual not for its content but for its creation. Medem, Inc. was founded by seven major medical groups: the American Medical Association, the American Academy of Pediatrics, The American College of Obstetricians and Gynecologists, the American Psychiatric Association, the American Academy of Ophthalmology, the American College of Allergy, Asthma & Immunology, and the American Society of Plastic Surgeons. These groups came together to try to provide authoritative medical information for physicians and patients alike. The site offers physicians an opportunity to provide information about their practices in a consistent format that makes it easy for patients to use. In addition, the site offers patients the American Medical Society's (AMA) "physician finder" service (Fig. 5.17). This service uses geographic information and the AMA's database of physicians to link up patients and practices.

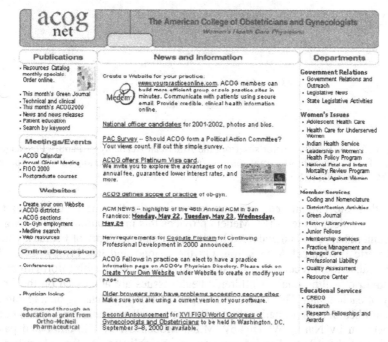

Figure 5.14. The American College of Obstetricians and Gynecologists makes use of its home page to provide information for both patients and members. With an appropriate password, members can access professional and other information. (**http://www.acog.org**)

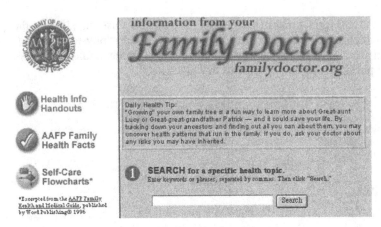

Figure 5.15. The Family Doctor site from the American Academy of Family Physicians offers fully searchable patient information also arranged by topic. (**http://www.familydoctor.org**)

At this site patients can sign up to receive the "Smart Parent's Health Source" newsletter (Fig. 5.18). Medem provides this information free of charge, with content supplied and endorsed by the American Academy of Pediatrics and the American Medical Association. On the second and last Fridays of each month, subscribers receive the latest pediatric news and health information in the pediatric health update. Children's health issues are addressed on the first Friday of each month. This includes in-depth information focusing on a featured children's health issue of national importance, as well as a children's health column written by Nancy W. Dickey, M.D., Medem's editor-in-chief and past president of the AMA. The information can be delivered to the subscriber's computer in either HTML or plain text formats. When signing up for this service, users can indicate areas of special interest for future topics. The site takes great care to address privacy and security issues, even going so far as to tell users why the subscription page asks the questions it does.

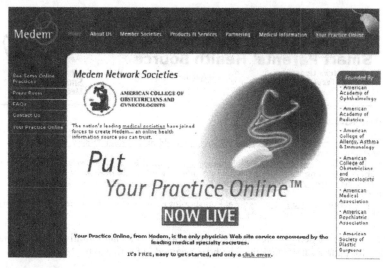

Figure 5.16. The Medem site (**http://www.medem.com**) was created by seven major medical groups including the American Medical Association.

Your Health

Medem is the only source for credible, comprehensive, and clinical healthcare information from both an individual's own physician and the nation's trusted medical societies.

Parents, sign up now for the Medem™ Smart Parents' Health Source newsletter! Click here to see previous issues.

Looking for a physician? Use the AMA Physician Finder!

AMA Physician Finder

Figure 5.17. At Medem, patients can sign up for electronic news letters or find physicians.

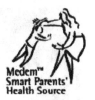

Welcome to Medem™
Smart Parents' Health Source

Pediatric News Update
Vol 1, Issue 1   August 11, 2000

In this issue...

- AAP Recommends Pneumococcal Vaccine for Children Younger Than 2 Years Old (New AAP policy statement)
- Air Bags May Cause Serious Eye Injuries in Children (New study from *Ophthalmology*)
- Tobacco Use Common Among College Students (New study from *JAMA*)
- Study Estimates 20% of SIDS Deaths Occur in Child Care Settings (New study from *Pediatrics*)
- AAP Recommends Ban on Corporal Punishment in Schools (New AAP policy statement)
- About Medem™ Smart Parents' Health Source

Figure 5.18. The Medem Smart Parents' Health Source is an authoritative source of information for patients and others that can be subscribed to for free at the Medem site.

An interesting sidelight on the Medem site is emerging as this book goes to press: It turns out that like so many of the .coms, a possibly flawed business plan, less than expected response from users and sponsors, and an operating cost of $1.5 million a month have resulted in financial disaster. There is a very real possibility of the project going under. There are some venture capital folks thinking about a bailout, but only if the involved organizations give up a great deal of their copyrighted material and 20% of their revenue-producing material as well. This material is what gives the site its veracity, but such a ceding would not be in the best interest of the organizations. As with other areas of electronic commerce, the outcome is yet to be determined.

The British philanthropic organization, the Wellcome Trust, supplies an excellent patient education and information site that includes pointers to current exhibits, news articles, and other forms of medical information not offered by the more text-based pages noted above (Fig. 5.19). Like sites offered by recognized specialty societies, this site carries with it the stamp of authority that can reassure patients that the information is mainstream, timely, and reliable. While often not well known outside of their own country, organizations such as the Wellcome trust or professional groups such as the American Medical Society can be readily found with common search engines. As with the Internet in general, the physical location of the computer server that holds the information is inconsequential and most often unknown to the end user. As mentioned above, except when national variations in drug availability or differing modes of medical practice come into play, the information that these sites contain should not be overlooked because of geographic or political boundaries.

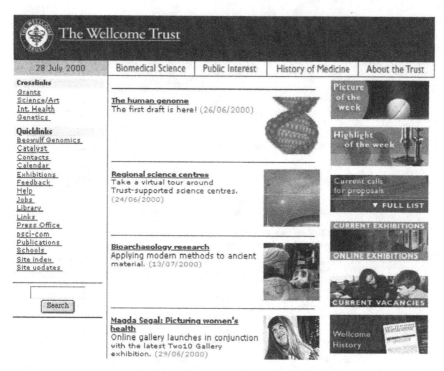

Figure 5.19. The British Wellcome Trust offers an excellent site for general health information and news. (**http://www.wellcome.ac.uk/**)

Direct Marketing

One relativly new phenomenon (a difficult concept in a field as new as the Internet) is that of the marketing of medical products and services directly to consumers. One does not even need a search engine to fine direct to consumer advertising for the latest drugs and devices. Major ethical pharmaceutical manufactures now introduce their new drugs with direct advertising and Web sites, even before providers have heard about the product. This can often mean that patients present to our offices requesting prescriptions for medications we have not heard about. As with much of today's advertising, these broadcast and print advertisements include the URL for the product's Web site. Some perceptive Web watchers have even learned to watch what site names companies are registering to get advanced information about corporate plans, mergers, and product introductions.

Examples of Web information sites about specific medicines (ethical and over the counter) abound and many are already familiar to anyone connected to the Internet. Less common, but growing, are sites marketing direct to consumer health-related goods and services. An example of this type of site is the one offered by "I am growing" (Fig. 5.20). This site offers to create a customized

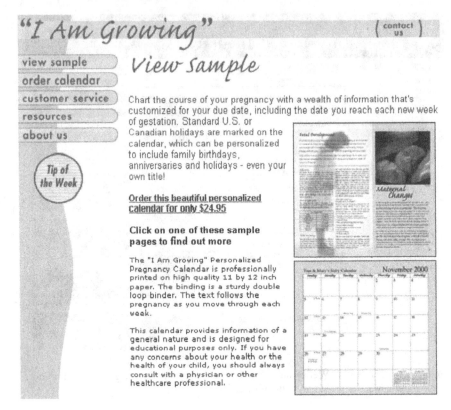

Figure 5.20. A growing number of companies offer medically related goods and services directly to consumers. This site offers customized pregnancy calendars. (**http://www.iamgrowing.com/**)

calendar for pregnant patients that gives them step-by-step information about the course of their pregnancy. Patients provide their due date and the calendar is customized for their particular pregnancy.

Finding Quality

With so many sites available, how do we guide our patients to information that can be trusted? Or, put another way, if I am a patient, whom can I trust? The most reliable first stop for any health information will be a site administered by a government agency or recognized professional society. While many times these sites may be obvious to us, our patients are less likely to automatically guess the proper agency or group. If there are sites that you find helpful, a list for your patients (printed or as links on a practice's Web page) can be a good way to avoid the pitfalls of bad information.

Sites offered by national societies dealing with specific disease states or conditions can be excellent sources of reliable information. The risk here is that there are many sites carrying names or logos that seem to be authoritative but are not. While it may be a bit of a judgment call, the National Society of Herbalists for Athlete's Foot and Related Diseases may not carry the same credibility as the American Academy of Dermatology (**http://www.aad.org/**). Often the distinctions are subtle and someone else may not recognize one person's authority. A very incomplete list of some organizational sites organized by topic or disease may be found in Appendix 2.

One effort to provide guidelines for the editorial content, advertising, privacy, and security for medical Internet sites has been the publication of standards by the American Medical Association (AMA). These guidelines have been instituted for all of the AMA Web sites and have been adopted by other sites as well. One subscriber to these standards is the Medem site (Fig. 5.16), though it should be remembered that Medem is a venture cofounded by the AMA and six other medical associations. While the AMA guidelines offer tools for judging the content of Internet sites, they do not intend to evaluate compliance or endorse sites based on these standards.

A group of health-related sites have banded together to provide some independent standards for Internet health sites. The Health on the Net (HON, Fig. 5.21) has posted these standards and provides a "seal of approval" for those sites that conform. This Swiss nonprofit corporation also offers visitors links and tools to integrate Web sites, journal articles, multimedia, and news for faster, richer search results. Also offered are links to MedLine and to a compilation of medically related image banks.

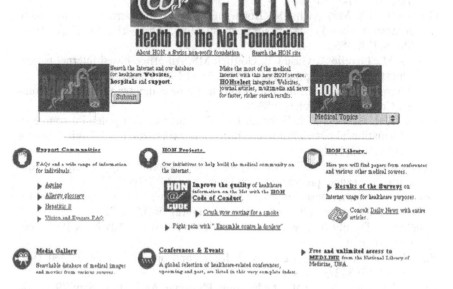

Figure 5.21. The Health On the Net Foundation attempts to provide standards for other health-related Internet sites. (**http://www.hon.ch/**)

Resources

Here is a (limited) list of references and sources of additional information about electronic patient education and information:

Bensen C, Stern J, Skinner E, et. al. An interactive, computer-based program to educate patients about genital herpes. Sex Transm Dis 1999 Jul;26(6):364-8.

Bergeron BP. Could your practice use a waiting room kiosk? How to turn waiting time into learning time. Postgrad Med 2000 Apr;107(4):41-3.

Bergeron BP. Technology-enabled education. Postgrad Med 1998 May;103(5):31-4.

Bergeron BP. Where to find practical patient education materials. Empowering your patients without spending a lot of time and money. Postgrad Med 1999 Nov;106(6):35-8.

Berridge E, Roudsari A, Taylor S, Carey S. Computer-aided learning for the education of patients and family practice professionals in the personal care of diabetes. Comput Methods Programs Biomed 2000 Jul;62(3):191-204.

Brennan PF. Health informatics and community health: support for patients as collaborators in care. Methods Inf Med 1999 Dec;38(4-5):274-8.

Dabney MK, Huelsman K. Counseling by computer: breast cancer risk and genetic testing. Developed by the University of Wisconsin—Madison Department of Medicine and the Program in Medical Ethics. Genet Test 2000;4(1):43-4.

Dausch JG, Golaszewski TJ. How to educate your patients. Internist 1992 Sep;33(8):31-3, 36.

Gustafson DH, McTavish FM, Boberg E, et al. Empowering patients using computer based health support systems. Qual Health Care 1999 Mar;8(1):49-56.

Helwig AL, Lovelle A, Guse CE, Gottlieb MS. An office-based Internet patient education system: a pilot study. J Fam Pract 1999 Feb;48(2):123-7.

Henchbarger TL. HMO health education enters the computer age. Healthc Comput Commun 1986 Jul;3(7):86-8.

Horton KM, Garland MR, Fishman EK. The Internet as a potential source of information about radiological procedures for patients. J Digit Imaging 2000 Feb;13(1):46-7.

Kolasa KM, Jobe AC, Miller MG. Using computer technology for nutrition education and cancer prevention. Acad Med 1996 May;71(5):525-6.

Lewis D. Computer-based approaches to patient education: a review of the literature. J Am Med Inform Assoc 1999 Jul-Aug;6(4):272-82.

Lyneham J. Twenty first century patient education. Aust J Adv Nurs 1999 Dec-Feb;17(2):29.

Patrick K. How patients use the web for second opinions. West J Med 1999 Jun;170(6):332-3. Review.

Rice NC. Guidelines for patient education. Physician Assist 1983 Sep;7(9):55-6.

Sefton E, Glazebrook C, Garrud P, Zaki I. Educating patients about malignant melanoma: computer-assisted learning in a pigmented lesion clinic. Br J Dermatol 2000 Jan;142(1):66-71.

Sheikh K. Computer-based support systems for women with breast cancer. JAMA 1999 Apr 14;281(14):1268-9.

Steinberg CS. Communicating with patients via e-mail: is it a good idea? J Am Optom Assoc 1999 Sep;70(9):599-601.

Stipp D. Health help on the Net. Fortune 1998 Jan 12;137(1):135-6.

Taylor K. The clinical e-mail explosion. Physician Exec 2000 Jan-Feb;26(1): 40-5.

6
Patient Care

As we have seen, the Internet has democratized the access to medical information. Patients have access to information (both good and bad) in ways and amounts never before possible. Patients who have access are potentially better informed—potentially even better informed than their health care provider. For the professional, the information transfer possible using the Internet can speed the distribution of new knowledge, enhance care, and ease the administrative tasks associated with the business of patient care.

The health care industry has been an early and aggressive user of computer and information management technologies, even before networks and the Internet became household commodities. One need look no further to find current examples of computers in medicine than the microprocessor-based pager or cell phone, the hospital information terminal where we get the results of computed tomography, or the security pad that lets us into the hospital after hours. The advent of easy-to-use browsers and the connectivity of the Internet make medical information current, easily accessed, and universally available. The Internet can also be the route to move specialized medical applications or remote medical information. Despite widespread use and enthusiasm, the value of computers and the Internet in most aspects of patient care has yet to be proved.

Diseases and Diagnosis Assistance

There is a vast amount of information available on the Internet that pertains to specific diseases or conditions. Access to this information can be useful to keep current with changing diagnostic or therapeutic options, or to aid in the diagnosis and management of uncommon conditions. The type of sites available range from those maintained by individuals (often with the disease or condition in question), organizations, or government agencies. The depth and reliability of information found are generally linked and increase with the size and credibility of the hosting organization. One example of the latter is the National Center for Biotechnology Information maintained by the National Library of Medicine (Fig. 6.1).

The importance of computerized information processing methods for the conduct of biomedical research was recognized in legislation that established the National Center for Biotechnology Information (NCBI) on November 4, 1988, as a division of the National Library of Medicine (NLM) at the National Institutes of Health (NIH). NLM was chosen because of its experience in creating and maintaining biomedical databases, and because as part of NIH it could establish an intramural research program in computational molecular biology. The NCBI was charged with creating automated systems for storing and analyzing knowledge about molecular biology, biochemistry, and genetics, as well as performing research into advanced methods of computer-based information

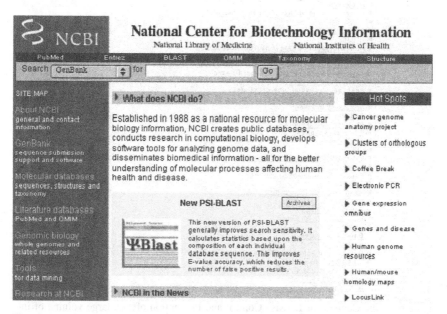

Figure 6.1. The National Center for Biotechnology Information Internet site offers links to the latest information about genetic and molecular diseases. (**http://www.ncbi. nlm.nih.gov**)

processing for analyzing the structure and function of biologically important molecules and compounds. They also coordinate efforts to gather biotechnology information worldwide through the use of the Internet and other methods. Their Internet site offers links to a large volume of innovative information about genetic and molecularly based diseases. They also provide educational resources and tools for data mining. This information is particularly useful when confronted with patients with inheritable diseases.

Another government site that has a wealth of disease-specific information is that maintained by the Centers for Disease Control and Prevention (Fig. 6.2). From the unusual to the urbane, this site offers authoritative information. Whether you are faced with an unusual patient or just a request for travel-related health precautions, this site can be invaluable.

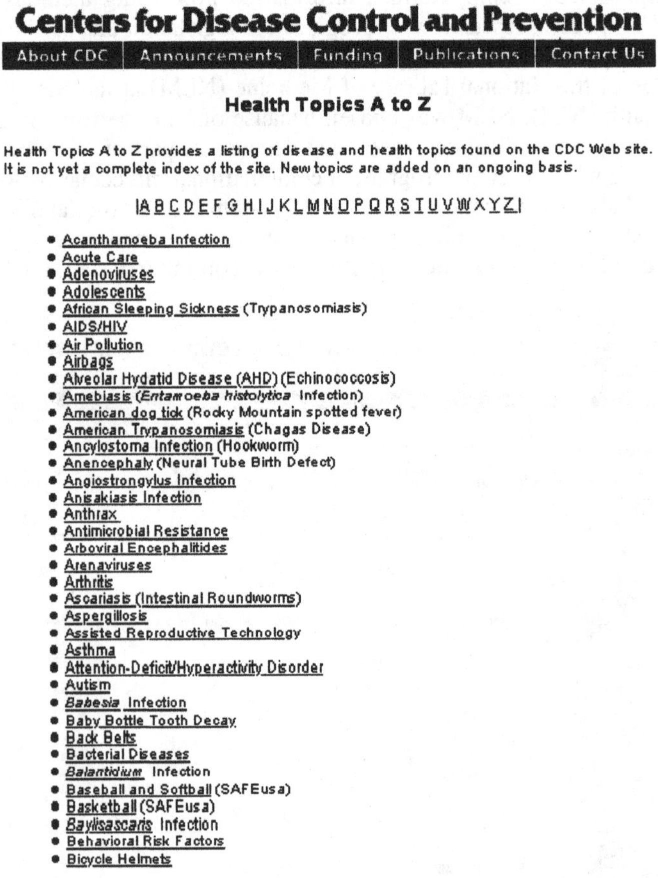

Centers for Disease Control and Prevention

| About CDC | Announcements | Funding | Publications | Contact Us |

Health Topics A to Z

Health Topics A to Z provides a listing of disease and health topics found on the CDC Web site. It is not yet a complete index of the site. New topics are added on an ongoing basis.

|A B C D E F G H I J K L M N O P Q R S T U V W X Y Z|

- Acanthamoeba Infection
- Acute Care
- Adenoviruses
- Adolescents
- African Sleeping Sickness (Trypanosomiasis)
- AIDS/HIV
- Air Pollution
- Airbags
- Alveolar Hydatid Disease (AHD) (Echinococcosis)
- Amebiasis (*Entamoeba histolytica* Infection)
- American dog tick (Rocky Mountain spotted fever)
- American Trypanosomiasis (Chagas Disease)
- Ancylostoma Infection (Hookworm)
- Anencephaly (Neural Tube Birth Defect)
- Angiostrongylus Infection
- Anisakiasis Infection
- Anthrax
- Antimicrobial Resistance
- Arboviral Encephalitides
- Arenaviruses
- Arthritis
- Ascariasis (Intestinal Roundworms)
- Aspergillosis
- Assisted Reproductive Technology
- Asthma
- Attention-Deficit/Hyperactivity Disorder
- Autism
- *Babesia* Infection
- Baby Bottle Tooth Decay
- Back Belts
- Bacterial Diseases
- *Balantidium* Infection
- Baseball and Softball (SAFEusa)
- Basketball (SAFEusa)
- *Baylisascaris* Infection
- Behavioral Risk Factors
- Bicycle Helmets

Figure 6.2. The Centers for Disease Control and Prevention offer a large volume of information about diseases and health-related topics accessible through an alphabetic listing. (**www.cdc.gov/health/diseases.htm**)

Research that Actually Helps

The volume of information that is available to health care providers has grown at a staggering rate. For graduates 10 years out from the completion of their residency, almost 90% of the medications and therapies available have been introduced after the completion of their training. How does the clinician sort out the information of significance from the background flurry of information crossing the door (or modem line) each day? One source for this type of assistance that is available on the Internet is the Cochran Library (Fig. 6.3).

The Cochrane Library grew out of the efforts of Archie Cochrane, a British epidemiologist, who recognized that people who want to make more informed decisions about health care do not have ready access to reliable reviews of the available evidence. In 1987, the year before Cochrane died, he referred to a systematic review of randomized controlled trials (RCTs) of care during pregnancy and childbirth as "a real milestone in the history of randomized trials and in the evaluation of care," and suggested that other specialties should copy the methods used. He suggested that if this was not done, important effects of health care (good and bad) would not be identified promptly, and people using the health services would be ill served. Without systematic, up-to-date reviews of previous research, plans for new research could not be well informed, and researchers and funding bodies might miss promising leads, and potentially embark on studies of questions that have already been answered.

Cochrane's suggestion that the methods used to prepare and maintain reviews of controlled trials in pregnancy and childbirth should be applied more widely was taken up by the Research and Development Programme, initiated to support the United Kingdom's National Health Service. Funds were provided to establish a "Cochrane Centre," to collaborate with others, in the UK and elsewhere, to facilitate systematic reviews of randomized controlled trials across all areas of health care. When the Cochrane Centre was opened, in Oxford, in October 1992,

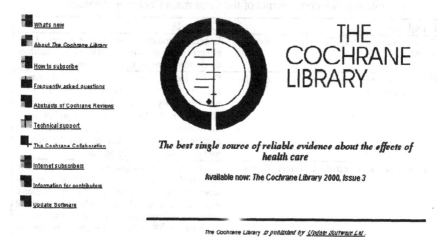

The best single source of reliable evidence about the effects of health care

Available now: The Cochrane Library 2000, Issue 3

The Cochrane Library is published by Update Software Ltd.

Figure 6.3. The Cochrane Library supplies a variety of analyses to support evidence-based medical practice. (**http://www.cochrane.org/cochrane/cdsr.htm**)

those involved expressed the hope that there would be a collaborative international response to Cochrane's agenda. This idea was outlined at a meeting organized six months later by the New York Academy of Sciences. In October 1993—at what was to become the first in a series of annual Cochrane Colloquia—77 people from eleven countries co-founded the Cochrane Collaboration.

Cochrane reviews (the principal output of the Collaboration) are published electronically in successive issues of the Cochrane Database of Systematic Reviews. These are available by subscription on the Internet or by CD-ROM, though the abstracts of Cochrane Reviews are available without charge and can be browsed or searched on the Internet. Preparation and maintenance of Cochrane reviews is the responsibility of international collaborative review groups. By the beginning of 1997, the existing and planned review groups (over 40) covered most of the important areas of health care. The members of these groups—researchers, health care professionals, consumers, and others—share an interest in generating reliable, up-to-date evidence relevant to the prevention, treatment, and rehabilitation of particular health problems or groups of problems. Their efforts have resulted in a rapidly growing collection of regularly updated, systematic reviews of the effects of health care. New reviews are added with each issue of the Cochrane Library. Cochrane reviews are reviews mainly of randomized controlled trials. Evidence is included or excluded on the basis of explicit quality criteria to minimize bias. Data are often combined statistically, with meta-analysis, to increase the power of the findings of numerous studies, each too small to produce reliable results individually. The components of the three main Cochrane databases are shown in Table 6.1. Publishing systematic reviews in an electronic form has great advantages over traditional methods: the reviews can be updated as new evidence emerges, and mistakes can be corrected in response to comments and criticisms. The review thereby continues to be the best single place where a distillation of the latest evidence is easily accessible.

Table 6.1 The components of the three main Cochrane databases

Database	Contents
The Cochrane Database of Systematic Reviews (CDSR)	Regularly updated, systematic reviews of the effects of health care, maintained by contributors to the Cochrane Collaboration.
Database of Abstracts of Reviews of Effectiveness (DARE)	DARE includes structured abstracts of systematic reviews from around the world, which have been critically appraised by reviewers at the NHS Centre for Reviews and Dissemination at the University of York, England. DARE also contains references to other reviews that may be useful for background information.
The Cochrane Controlled Trials Register (CCTR)	CCTR is a bibliography of controlled trials identified by contributors to the Cochrane Collaboration and others, as part of an international effort to hand search the world's journals and create an unbiased source of data for systematic reviews. CCTR includes reports published in conference proceedings and in many other sources not currently listed in MEDLINE or other bibliographic databases.

Access to the Cochrane databases is by subscription, though the abstracts are available without charge through their Internet site. At the time of this writing, the cost for a full subscription is $125 for one year's access. There are some minor differences between the servers located in the United States and the United Kingdom, though these are not of practical significance.

Another Internet site that is devoted to applying research data to develop evidence-based medical practice is supplied by the School of Health and Related Research (ScHARR), in Sheffield, UK (Fig. 6.4). ScHARR is one of the four schools in the faculty of medicine at the University of Sheffield. ScHARR is a significant university-based concentration of health-related data in Trent and one of the most important in the UK. This easy to navigate site has an extensive list of links and resources for finding, appraising, and implementing current research findings. Resources for software, journals, databases, and organizations are well represented, easy to find, accurate, and current.

If you or your patients want information about ongoing clinical trials, the ClinicalTrials.gov site should be considered (Fig. 6.5). This site was developed as a collaboration between the National Institutes of Health and the National Library of Medicine. ClinicalTrials.gov was developed to provide patients, family members, and members of the public current information about clinical research studies. While this site is geared mainly toward interested lay surfers and study participants, physicians can find useful information about ongoing studies. You can find information about specific research based on condition or sponsor, or you can do a specialized search by disease, location, or treatment. The site offers links to MedLine and NIH health information site.

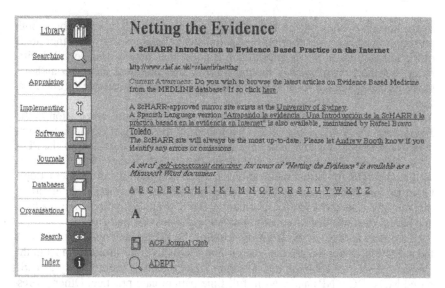

Figure 6.4. The School of Health and Related Research (ScHARR), in Sheffield, UK, offers a large number of resources for applying current research data in the clinical setting. (**http://www.shef.ac.uk/~scharr/ir/netting/**)

ClinicalTrials.gov

A service of the National Institutes of Health
Developed by the National Library of Medicine   *Linking Patients to Medical Research*

| Home | Search | Browse | Resources | Help | What's New | About |

The U.S. National Institutes of Health, through its National Library of Medicine, has developed *ClinicalTrials.gov* to provide patients, family members and members of the public current information about clinical research studies. Before searching, you may want to learn more about clinical trials and more about this Web site. Check often for regular updates to *ClinicalTrials.gov*.

Search Clinical Trials
Enter words or phrases, separated by commas:

[   ]   [Search] Tips

Search by Specific Information
Focused Search - search by disease, location, treatment, sponsor...

Browse
Browse by Condition - studies listed by disease or condition
Browse by Sponsor - studies listed by funding organization

Resource Information
Understanding Clinical Trials - information explaining and describing clinical trials
MEDLINE*plus* - health care information selected by the National Library of Medicine
NIH Health Information - research supported by the National Institutes of Health
healthfinder® - consumer health and human services information

Figure 6.5. The ClinicalTrials.gov site answers questions about currently ongoing clinical trials and clinical research in general.

Drugs and Prescribing

There are many sites on the Internet that can provide information about both prescription and nonprescription medications and therapies. As with other areas of the Internet, most of this information is good, but some is of uncertain legitimacy. For the busy physician, the most useful sites are those that offer authoritative, broad coverage so that the information needed is available in one location.

For many practitioners, the main source of clinical drug information is the *Physicians' Desk Reference* (PDR) published by the Medical Economics Company. This same company makes available the electronic equivalent of the PDR on its Web site (Fig. 6.6). This site offers the *Physicians' Desk Reference* as well as the PDR for herbal medications and PDR for multiple drug interactions. Other options include access to new drug and pricing information. In addition, the site offers medical news, information about what our patients are reading, and access to controlled-circulation journals published by the firm.

To obtain access to the electronic form of the PDR, users must register with the site. Registration is free but free on-line access to drug information from the *Physicians' Desk Reference* and *Stedman's Dictionary* is granted only to U.S.-based MDs, DOs, NPs and PAs in full-time patient care practice. Other professionals or consumers wishing to access these particular features on-line may subscribe on-line for $9.95/month or $99.95/year. Once you have registered, you may search the indices of the *Physicians' Desk Reference* to find a drug by product name, manufacturer, product category, indication, contraindication, side effect, or drug interaction. Recently approved drugs may not be integrated into this database, as the information available tends to reflect the information contained in the current print version. You may also search the full text of the *Physicians' Desk Reference* and of the PDR addenda, which contain the monographs of recently approved drugs.

In addition to the databases of prescription medications familiar to most practitioners, the PDR site also offers the searchable information from the PDR for herbal medicines. This area of medicine has long been overlooked by compilations and textbooks, making it difficult to find information when it is needed. While there is often limited information known about the actual action and uses of many herbal products, this database allows users to search by name, category, indication, or side effects. The site also has photos of many of the bioactive plants used in making these treatments. This can be useful when trying to identify the source of a hypersensitivity or a contact allergy. The site can be very useful if the herbal product you are looking for is one that is listed. The interface is not efficient and seemingly common agents are missing. A search for "Don Quai" (a commonly used agent for menstrual pain—*Angelica Sinsensis*)

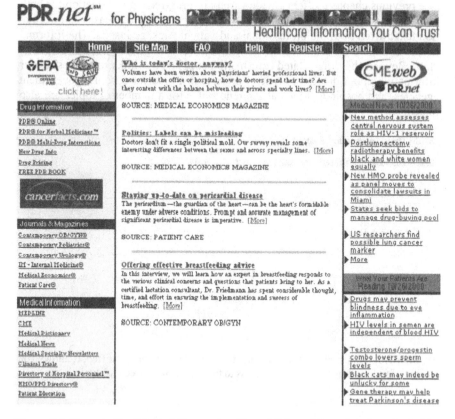

Figure 6.6. Presented by Medical Economics (the publisher of the printed version), this site offers the *Physicians' Desk Reference* (PDR) as well as the PDR for herbal medications and PDR multidrug interactions. (**http://physician.pdr.net/physician/ index.htm**)

could not locate any information by common name, scientific name, or indication.

A particularly useful aspect of this site is the page that allows you to enter a number of drugs and determine whether they may interact with one another or are contraindicated (Fig. 6.7). This interactive ability to test for possible problems of drug therapy is not readily available elsewhere, making this function worth the time taken to register. To use this function, medications are selected from alphabetic lists or searched for by trade or generic name. Once the patient's medication list has been completed, clicking on the start check button returns a listing of interactions or other pertinent information. Using the interface requires clicking on a number of pages to navigate through the list of drugs available. While you can edit (delete from) the list of drugs you have compiled, you cannot type in the drugs directly. This results in a minimum of two pages of displays for each drug—more if your drugs occur late in an alphabetic listing or there are several drugs that contain the agent of interest.

Another useful Internet source for drug-related information is the Drug InfoNet site (Fig. 6.8). This private Health On the Net Foundation subscriber (see previous chapter), offers a wide variety of drug-related information for both providers and patients alike. The site contains searchable databases of information taken from both the professional and patient package inserts. The information is available by brand name, generic name, manufacturer, and therapeutic class. Beyond the drug-related information supplied are links to other sites for information about diseases, medical news items, medical schools, government agencies, and hospitals. Medical reference sites for a number of topics are also linked.

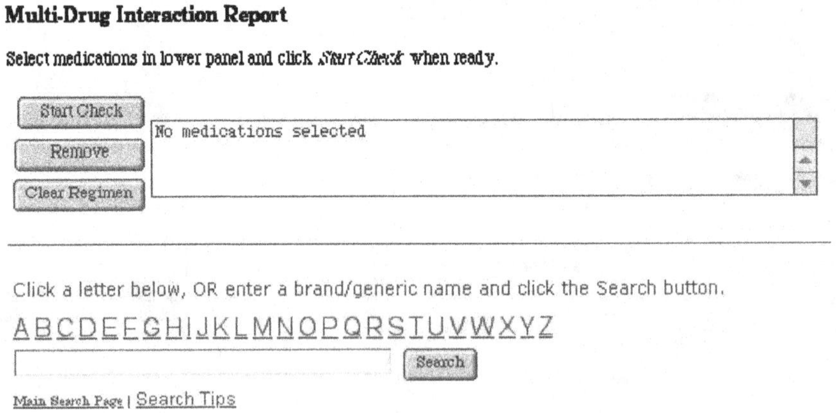

Multi-Drug Interaction Report

Select medications in lower panel and click *Start Check* when ready.

Start Check	No medications selected
Remove	
Clear Regimen	

Click a letter below, OR enter a brand/generic name and click the Search button.

A B C D E F G H I J K L M N O P Q R S T U V W X Y Z

[   ] [Search]

Main Search Page | Search Tips

Figure 6.7. Available at the PDR.net site, the Multi-Drug Interaction Report allows you to check for drug-drug interactions. Access to this site requires free registration.

Drug InfoNet

THE INTERNET SOURCE FOR HEALTHCARE INFORMATION

Drug Information

Disease Information

Ask The Doctor

FAQ'S

Pharmaceutical
    Manufacturer Info

Healthcare News

Health Information

Healthcare Org. Sites

Government Sites

Medical Reference
    & Study

Hospitals On-line

Med Schools On-Line

Drug InfoNet is your one-stop WWW site for all your healthcare informational needs. We provide both information and links to areas on the web concerning healthcare and pharmaceutical-related topics. This free service is brought to you to improve your education as consumers and healthcare professionals.

SEARCH Drug InfoNet!

[Search]

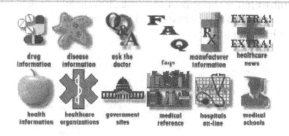

drug
information

disease
information

ask the
doctor

faqs

manufacturer
information

healthcare
news

health
information

healthcare
organizations

government
sites

medical
reference

hospitals
on-line

medical
schools

Figure 6.8. Supplied by Drug InfoNet, Inc. this site offer connections to patient and professional package insert information as well as other useful drug and general medical information links. (**http://www.druginfonet.com/**)

An extensive site offering information on almost any aspect of pharmacy and pharmaceuticals is the Martindale's Health Science Guide located at **www-sci.lib.uci.edu/HSG/Pharmacy.html#PC3**. This site offers international information about drugs and companies and is very useful when patients travel to or from other regions. The site contains drug databases, disease tutorials, and specialized calculators. From Chinese herbal medicine to time zone information, a global wave model, or a ship's schedules, you can probably find it here. Drug information at this site is available in six different languages—a useful attribute if you need to provide information to a foreign patient or colleague.

One aspect of pharmaceuticals and the Internet that is of concern to professionals and consumers alike is Internet prescribing and prescription fulfillment. The availability of prescription drugs on-line without a prescription has become a national and international issue resulting in congressional hearings and new laws. For most honest individuals, particularly the home-bound or elderly, the option to fill their physician's prescription this way could be an advantage. Unfortunately, it is not always possible to tell if the pharmacy you have found through the Internet is a legitimate licensed and inspected pharmacy. In response to these concerns, the National Association of Boards of Pharmacy (NABP) developed the Verified Internet Pharmacy Practice Sites (VIPPS) program to provide a "seal of approval" to those sites that meet specific criteria and pass an onsite inspection. A coalition of state and federal regulatory agencies, professional associations, and consumer advocacy groups were involved in establishing the criteria used for this certification process. Those who meet these criteria can display the VIPPS logo and can be verified with the NABP through a linked site (**www.nabp.net**, Fig. 6.9). Pharmacies certified by this program are licensed by each state to which they dispense, thus avoiding the question of serving patients across state lines, an issue that has not been clearly resolved when it comes to medical practice (see Chapter 10).

Patients should be advised that sites that are of greatest concerns for licensure, inspection, or legal problems are those that advertise prescription drugs (or their "nonprescription equivalents") used to enhance "lifestyles." These sites offer drugs to enhance sexual desire or performance, treat male pattern baldness, or promote weight loss. There are even sites that promote controlled substances or chemicals commonly abused by teens and young adults. Some of these sites attempt to avoid United States laws by being located in foreign countries and it is often difficult to tell when this is the case. Physicians should take a lead in advising patients about the risks associated with such sites. Some general guidelines are shown in Table 6.2.

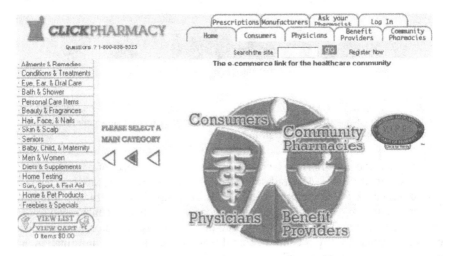

Figure 6.9. The Clickpharmacy.com site is an example of an Internet pharmacy site that displays the VIPPS seal and endorsement. (**www.clickpharmacy.com**)

Table 6.2. General guidelines for using on-line prescription sites

- Don't purchase drugs from sites that offer to prescribe a drug for the first time without a physical examination, sell a prescription drug without a prescription, or sell drugs that are not FDA approved.
- Don't purchase drugs from a site that does not offer access to a licensed pharmacist who can answer questions. This can be important for patients taking multiple medications or have medication allergies that need to consult the pharmacist before starting a new prescription.
- Don't deal with any site that does not specifically identify itself and provide contact addresses or phone numbers. These would be needed if a problem or question should arise.
- Avoid any site that offers "new" or "quick" cures to serious disorders. If you are looking for miracles, check the religion site of your choice.
- Avoid sites that use unnecessary jargon or impressive terminology—this may be an effort to hide the lack of substance or validity.
- Avoid sites that claim the medical or scientific community is suppressing them (or the products they offer). There is no cure for cancer that the medical community is trying to suppress. (There may be one for obesity, but that is a different story…)
- Avoid sites that use case histories, patient testimonials, or reports of dramatic cures—legitimate sites and products do not need this type of hype.
- Don't deal with any site that refuses a request for licensure information. All states require the licensure of pharmacists and pharmacies before they are allowed to provide prescription drugs. In the case of 40 states, this is true if they do business in the state even though they are physically located outside the state's borders. If the site can't (or won't) provide the information, don't deal with them.

Medical Record Keeping

Several companies offer electronic medical record systems that are either stand-alone or Internet based. These systems are intended to replace the medical record made during patient encounters, but they are generally limited to patient care in only a few specialties. Electronic medical records offer legibility, accessibility, and the ability to provide dynamic suggestions about management, billing, or emerging problems as care progresses. These systems can interact with a hospital or laboratory information system, a radiology file system, or other source of patient information to make accessible pertinent information needed for patient care. Many systems interact directly with computerized scheduling and billing systems to provide an integrated office management tool. An example of this type of system is Logician marketed by Medscape (Fig. 6.10).

In most cases, electronic records systems are based on prestructured forms of encounter with fill-in blanks, buttons, and check boxes or pull-down options to construct the record of the appointment (Fig. 6.11). In some cases, the templates are extensively prewritten and all that remains is to click on selected text to make modifications (Fig. 6.12). When this path is taken, the modifiable text or information is presented in a different color, typeface, or font.

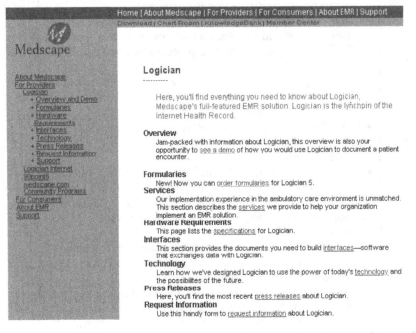

Figure 6.10. The Logician system of medical records offered by Medscape can be toured with a description and demonstration at the Medscape Web site. (**www.medicalogic.com/products/logician/index.html?id=hompro#**)

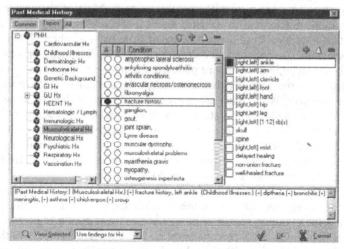

Figure 6.11. Check boxes, radio buttons, pull-down menus, or fill-in blanks allows electronic medical records to be modified to reflect the patient encounter. This example is from the Charting Plus 4 system from Medinotes. (**http://www.medinotes.com**)

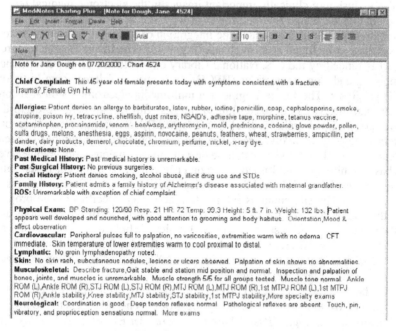

Figure 6.12. Some electronic medical records use templates with text that can be modified as needed. This example is from the Charting Plus 4 system. (**www.medinotes.com**)

Some electronic medical record systems will suggest appropriate billing codes or make recommendations about additional elements necessary to support billing for a given level of service. Other systems offer physician referral letters, patient instructions, and superbill modules as well. Most of the systems currently available are limited to specific medical specialties. They work well if you practice in one of these areas, but are of little use elsewhere. Even within covered specialties, newer or less common conditions, diagnoses, or treatments may not be included in the standard package. Changes may be made by the user or supplied from the provider, but this makes the system less convenient and more user intensive. While there are many satisfied users of these systems, there have not been any systematic studies to show that they save either time or money over paper records. The choice to use an electronic medical record must be individualized and based on the skills, needs, specialty, and volume of the practice. Examples, demonstrations, additional information, and frequently asked questions are available at a number of Internet sites.

Many of these systems use local intranets or the Internet to transmit or store the medical records. In some cases, the system uses these communication channels to pass the evolving record of the encounter from person to person within the office, before the encounter is complete and the record stored. With these systems, the record begins with the scheduling of the patient's appointment. The record is updated when the patient checks in, the nurse is notified, and intake information and vital signs are entered. The physician encounter is documented, and the record completed with the patient's checkout and departure.

The inclusion of clinically important images in the electronic medical record is the goal of the Image Engine project of the Clinical Multimedia Laboratory. Information about this project and the integration of images in an electronic record system can be found at its Web site (Fig. 6.13). The Image Engine research project is funded by the U.S. National Library of Medicines' High Performance Computing and Communications (HPCC) and National Telemedicine Initiative (NTI) programs. The Image Engine is a multimedia electronic medical record system that integrates digitized clinical images with textual data stored in the University of Pittsburgh Medical Center's MARS electronic medical record system. The project involves research and development in a number of areas including clinical multimedia database design, image compression, client-server database architecture, multimedia computer-user interfaces, agent-based integration and retrieval of clinical data, medical vocabularies, and Internet access to medical data. The site contains information about the specifics of the project, sites that are currently using the system, and a compilation of presentations and publications about the system and related topics. A link to specifics about the chart engine medical records system is under development. Examples of the types of images that can be included in the medical record are shown in a database of sample images (Fig. 6.14).

For those interested in the current state of the development for electronic medical records, the National Academy Press offers on-line access to the revised edition of *The Computer-Based Patient Record: An Essential Technology for Health Care* at **http://www.nap.edu/catalog/5306.html**. At this site, you can choose to purchase the book, view the text on line, or view summaries of the information.

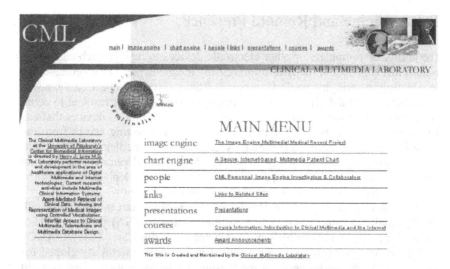

Figure 6.13. The Clinical Multimedia Laboratory at the University of Pittsburgh Medical Center hosts this site that contains information about the integration of clinical images in an electronic medical record system. (**http://www.cml.upmc.edu/**)

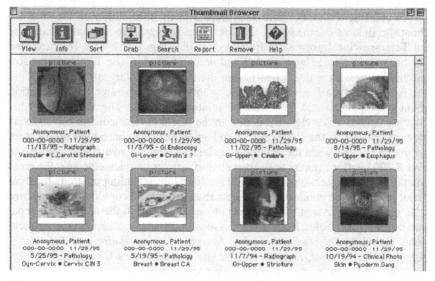

Figure 6.14. The Clinical Multimedia Laboratory site includes examples of the type of images that someday may be part of an electronic medical record. (**http://www.cml.upmc.edu/cml/imageengine/sampleImages.html**)

Telemedicine and Remote Presence

The ability of computers or other electronic devices to rapidly exchange information has engendered the rise in interest in "telemedicine." Telemedicine has been defined as bringing medical resources from a distance to bear on the needs of the patient at hand. This can be as simple as paging a chief resident to come to your assistance with a deteriorating patient or as complex as devices that can assess and transmit the vital signs of a patient who is sitting across from the television set in his home. In common usage, today's telemedicine means a bidirectional exchange of medically important data. The telephone was the first pathway for this type of exchange and connections to the telephone network (by computers) remains a common part of the systems in place now.

High-speed exchange of medical information got its start in the 1960s with the National Aeronautics and Space Administration (NASA) program "Space Technology Applied to Rural Papago Advanced Health Care" (STARPAHC). This program sought to apply the medical monitoring systems developed for space travel to the health needs of the Papago Indian reservation. Used as a test of feasibility rather than a cost-effective solution, the STARPAHC project showed both the possibilities and limitations of the available technology. As bandwidth (the ability to send large amounts of data rapidly) has increased, great strides have occurred in development and implementation of telemedicine.

As you might expect, there is a great deal of information on the Internet about the field of telemedicine. One of the most extensive and authoritative is the Telemedicine Information Exchange (TIE) (Fig. 6.15). The Telemedicine Information Exchange was created and is maintained by the Telemedicine Research Center with major support from the National Library of Medicine. This site is a comprehensive, international, quality-filtered resource for information about telemedicine and telemedicine-related activities. The site offers a bimonthly column covering what is new in the world of telemedicine and an overview of updates to the Web page. You can subscribe to an e-mail notification service to tell you when the column is updated. There is a searchable database of over 8,700 citations (many with abstracts) of articles on telemedicine—the most comprehensive collection of telemedicine literature including citations from all major telemedicine publications. The database is updated continuously and there is an on-line submission form for users to add citations to the database. A separate section for articles from current issues of all major telemedicine publications, including *Telemedicine Today, Journal of Telemedicine and Telehealth, Telemedicine Journal*, and others. The site also maintains lists of current telemedicine programs, meetings, and funding opportunities.

For those active in the field of telemedicine or exploring the options, the TIE site offers a collection of news, citations, articles, and specific links to legal issues and barriers to telemedicine, such as licensure and reimbursement. There is also a list of current legislation affecting telemedicine. A directory of 170 vendors of telemedicine equipment, searchable by company name, geographic location, or product category, is also found at this versatile site. Besides the expected links to other telemedicine sites, there are also sections devoted to job opportunities (with the ability to add your own listing) and basic information on how to

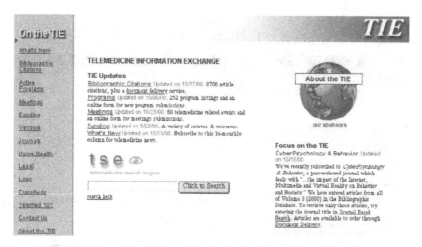

Figure 6.15. The Telemedicine Information Exchange is a serious resource for the professional or interested consumer. (**http://tie.telemed.org/**)

start a telemedicine program. The TIE site is another Health on the Net subscriber site.

Another site of primary interest to telemedicine professionals, but of some interest to physicians and health consumers in general, is the site maintained by the American Telemedicine Association (**http://www.atmeda.org**). Established in 1993 as a nonprofit organization and headquartered in Washington, DC, membership in the association is open to individuals, companies, and other organizations with an interest in promoting the deployment of telemedicine throughout the United States and worldwide. The site offers a members-only side and a public side, including a yet to be implemented section on "e-health."

The National Library of Medicine (NLM) maintains a site devoted to the National Telemedicine Initiative (Fig. 6.16). The National Telemedicine Initiative was announced in 1996 to fund 19-multiyear projects aimed at assessing the implementation and use of telemedicine technologies. The projects funded affect rural, inner city, and suburban areas and evaluate the use of telemedicine in a variety of settings. Two additional projects were announced in September 1997. The NLM site provides information about the National Telemedicine Initiative itself, projects supported by the initiative, and upcoming meetings. Links are provided to other sites supported by the initiative as well as resources of interest to the telemedicine professional. For the telemedicine novice, the site can give a good overview of the field and connections to demonstration projects and results that give an idea of current capabilities and future directions. This includes information about foreign telemedicine projects as well.

For those who are active in the field of telemedicine (or just want to keep up with the field) there is the new on-line magazine *Telemedicine Today* (**http://www.telemedtoday.com**). Working with several of the main organizations involved with telemedicine and electronic medical applications, *Telemedicine Today* carries articles and news of interest to the telemedicine community. Paper subscriptions are available for $125 for one year or $199 for two (at the

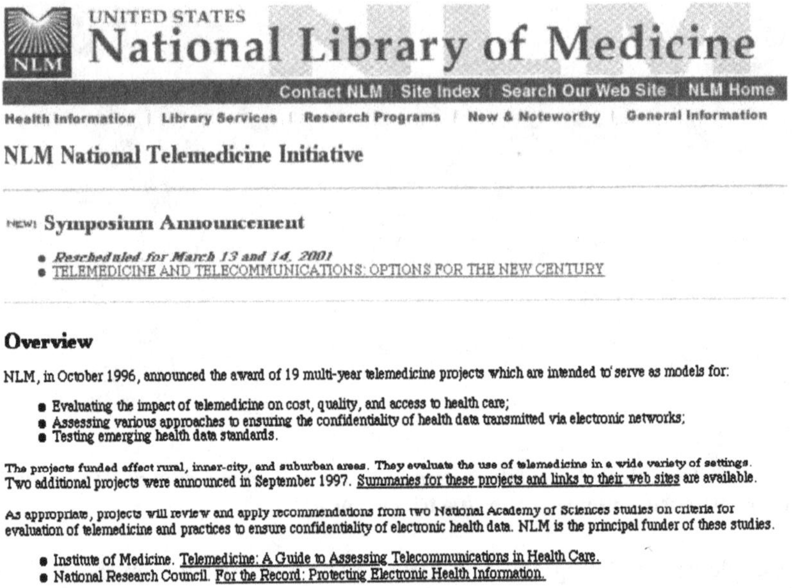

UNITED STATES
NLM
National Library of Medicine

Contact NLM | Site Index | Search Our Web Site | NLM Home

Health Information | Library Services | Research Programs | New & Noteworthy | General Information

NLM National Telemedicine Initiative

NEW! Symposium Announcement

- *Rescheduled for March 13 and 14, 2001*
- TELEMEDICINE AND TELECOMMUNICATIONS: OPTIONS FOR THE NEW CENTURY

Overview

NLM, in October 1996, announced the award of 19 multi-year telemedicine projects which are intended to serve as models for:

- Evaluating the impact of telemedicine on cost, quality, and access to health care;
- Assessing various approaches to ensuring the confidentiality of health data transmitted via electronic networks;
- Testing emerging health data standards.

The projects funded affect rural, inner-city, and suburban areas. They evaluate the use of telemedicine in a wide variety of settings. Two additional projects were announced in September 1997. Summaries for these projects and links to their web sites are available.

As appropriate, projects will review and apply recommendations from two National Academy of Sciences studies on criteria for evaluation of telemedicine and practices to ensure confidentiality of electronic health data. NLM is the principal funder of these studies.

- Institute of Medicine. Telemedicine: A Guide to Assessing Telecommunications in Health Care.
- National Research Council. For the Record: Protecting Electronic Health Information.

Figure 6.16. The National Library of Medicine maintains this site for information about the National Telemedicine Initiative. (**http://www.nlm.nih.gov/research/telemedinit.html**)

time of this writing), but samples may be requested and feature articles may be accessed on-line free. One unusual aspect of this site is the Digital studio where features and interviews are available as Real Video files that can be downloaded and played on the user's computer. Like other video information, the data files involved are large, so that without a very fast connection users will encounter long download times or jumpy, interrupted feeds when the data are viewed in real time. Video files are available in nine different categories ranging from features to telepsychiatry.

Resources

Here is a (limited) list of references and sources of additional information about electronic patient care:

Bensen C, Stern J, Skinner E, Beutner K, et al. An interactive, computer-based program to educate patients about genital herpes. Sex Transm Dis. 1999;26:364.

Cochrane AL. Effectiveness and Efficiency. Random Reflections on Health Services. London: Nuffield Provincial Hospitals Trust, 1972. (Reprinted in 1989 in association with the BMJ)

Cochrane AL. 1931-1971: a critical review, with particular reference to the medical profession. In: Medicines for the Year 2000. London: Office of Health Economics, 1979, 1-11.

Dick RS, Steen EB, Detmer DE, eds, Committee on Improving the Patient Record, Institute of Medicine. The Computer-Based Patient Record: An Essential Technology for Health Care, Revised Edition. Washington, DC: National Academy Press, 1997.

Lindberg DA, Humphreys BL. Computers in medicine. JAMA. 1995;273:1667.

National Library of Medicine. Current Bibliographies in Medicine: Telemedicine: Past, Present, Future. CBM. 1995;95-3.

Paperny DM. Computers and information technology: implications for the 21st century. Adolesc Med. 2000;11:183.

Smith R. Computers in medicine: searching for the rainbow and the pot of gold. Br Med J 1982;284:1859.

Strode SW. Gustke S, Allen A. Technical and clinical progress in telemedicine. JAMA. 1999;281:1066.

7

Medical Literature, Publishing and Informatics

We think of the Internet in terms of spinning logos and spectacular graphics, but until recently it was completely text based—it was a system only a "computer geek" could love. Consequently, it should be no surprise that the Internet is most efficient at transmitting text. Text is compact information that requires only the most basic conventions for translation. In fact, the translation standard that is used (ASCII) was developed for the Teletype industry long before the Web left the province of the arachnids. For this reason, publishing (medical or otherwise) has been intimately intertwined with the Web from its beginning.

Publishing and the Web

Publishers were some of the first to use intranets to exchange text files between the computers of writers, editors, compositors, typesetters, and printers. This allowed for speed, streamlining, and the elimination of some intermediate steps along the way. It was only a small step to involve the Internet. What has been a fundamental change, however, has been the inclusion of outsiders (authors and users) in these systems. Today, information supplied across the Internet allows authors to submit articles directly, publishers to skip typesetting, and users to access information in ways never before possible. Access to the full text of journals and other publications is common. Novels may be downloaded in seconds and read in electronic books while commuting. (Hopefully on public transportation rather than while behind the wheel.) In medicine, it has been the publishing of journal information that has most profoundly been affected.

Information for Authors

Many medical journals now offer information for potential authors on their Web sites or through those of their sponsoring organizations (Fig. 7.1). While traditionally published somewhere in the first issue of each volume, the electronic versions of this information are readily located and accessed when needed. Not only do these lists provide an author with the style the journal editors expect, they outline the submission requirements that must be met for an article to be considered. In many cases, the journal will also provide the checklist that must accompany either paper or electronic submissions for consideration (Fig. 7.2).

One of the most extensive collections of information on medical publishing is maintained by the Raymon H. Mulford Library at the Medical College of Ohio (Fig. 7.3). This site is invaluable as a resource for anyone wishing to publish in a medical journal. The site has links to specific information for authors and the submission requirements for essentially all of the major and minor medical journals. Here you will find links to Web sites with instructions to authors for over 3,000 journals in the health and life sciences. All links are to "primary sources," that is to publishers or organizations with editorial responsibilities for the titles. Consequently, there is no outdated information and no blind leads to follow. In addition, the site provides links to information

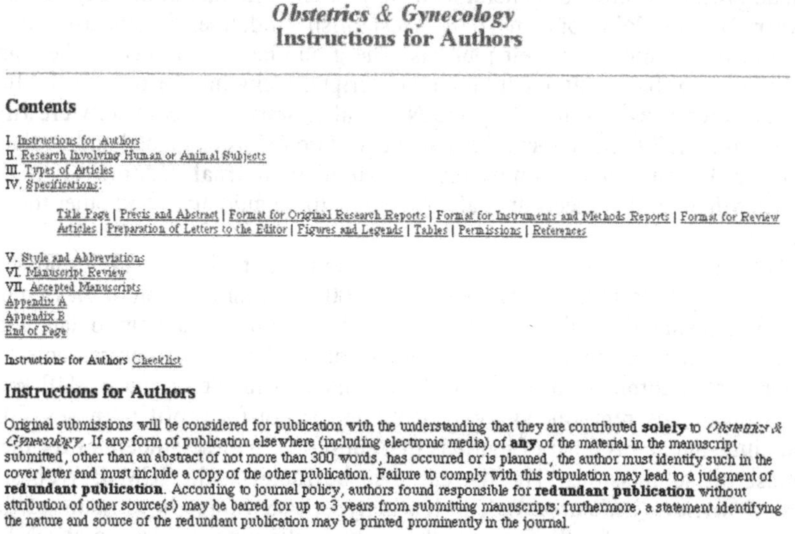

Obstetrics & Gynecology
Instructions for Authors

Contents

I. Instructions for Authors
II. Research Involving Human or Animal Subjects
III. Types of Articles
IV. Specifications:

Title Page | Précis and Abstract | Format for Original Research Reports | Format for Instruments and Methods Reports | Format for Review Articles | Preparation of Letters to the Editor | Figures and Legends | Tables | Permissions | References

V. Style and Abbreviations
VI. Manuscript Review
VII. Accepted Manuscripts
Appendix A
Appendix B
End of Page

Instructions for Authors Checklist

Instructions for Authors

Original submissions will be considered for publication with the understanding that they are contributed **solely** to *Obstetrics & Gynecology*. If any form of publication elsewhere (including electronic media) of **any** of the material in the manuscript submitted, other than an abstract of not more than 300 words, has occurred or is planned, the author must identify such in the cover letter and must include a copy of the other publication. Failure to comply with this stipulation may lead to a judgment of **redundant publication**. According to journal policy, authors found responsible for **redundant publication** without attribution of other source(s) may be barred for up to 3 years from submitting manuscripts; furthermore, a statement identifying the nature and source of the redundant publication may be printed prominently in the journal.

Figure 7.1. Elsevier publishing (publishers of the journal *Obstetrics & Gynecology*, shown here) offer detailed instructions for authors at their Web site. (**http://www-east.elsevier.com/ong/fullinst.htm**)

Obstetrics & Gynecology
Instructions for Authors

A completed Checklist and Agreement must accompany each manuscript submitted to *Obstetrics & Gynecology*.
A photocopy of these forms may be used. Submissions lacking a completed checklist and agreement will be returned to the sender. Full Instructions for Authors are provided in the January and July issues.

Checklist

General

_____ Two complete sets of the manuscript (including tables) are submitted.

_____ Manuscript is typed double-spaced, with ample, left-justified, margins.

_____ Pages are numbered consecutively, starting with the title page; the author's last name is typed in the top right corner of each page.

_____ Only standard abbreviations are included.

Title Page

_____ On the first page are typed the title, author name(s) and major degree(s), affiliation(s), and the source(s) of funding for the work or study.

Figure 7.2. Many journals supply the required submission checklist on-line in printable format. The example shown is for the journal *Obstetrics & Gynecology*. (**http://www-east.elsevier.com/ong/checklist.htm**)

needed for medical research and publishing in general. The site could not be easier to use, with information organized by the title of the journal and handy jumps from the top of the page to each alphabetic section. General information sites and those of broad interest are located at the head of the list.

One of the general information links offered by the Mulford site is to the Uniform Requirements for Manuscripts Submitted to Biomedical Publications; otherwise known as the "Vancouver Style." This consensus on style grew out of a small group of editors of general medical journals who met informally in Vancouver, British Columbia, in 1978 to establish guidelines for the format of manuscripts submitted to their journals. The group became known as the Vancouver Group. Its requirements for manuscripts, including formats for bibliographic references developed by the National Library of Medicine, were first published in 1979. Since then, the Vancouver Group has expanded and evolved into the International Committee of Medical Journal Editors (ICMJE, **www.icmje.org**) that meets annually to review these guidelines and other topics of concern.

The entire Uniform Requirements document was revised in 1997 and sections were updated in May 1999 and May 2000. A major revision of these standards is scheduled for 2001 and this is a good site to use to stay up to date with the requirement changes. The total content of the Uniform Requirements for Manuscripts Submitted to Biomedical Journals is available on the ICMJE Web site and may be reproduced for educational or not-for-profit purposes. The committee maintains a list of journals that subscribe to these guidelines for their manuscript submissions. The list can also be found at the ICMJE Web site (**www.icmje.org/jrnlist.html**). The list is hyperlinked directly to many of the Internet home sites for the journals themselves, allowing the user to check for use of the Vancouver style and jump directly to the publisher's site for more specific details.

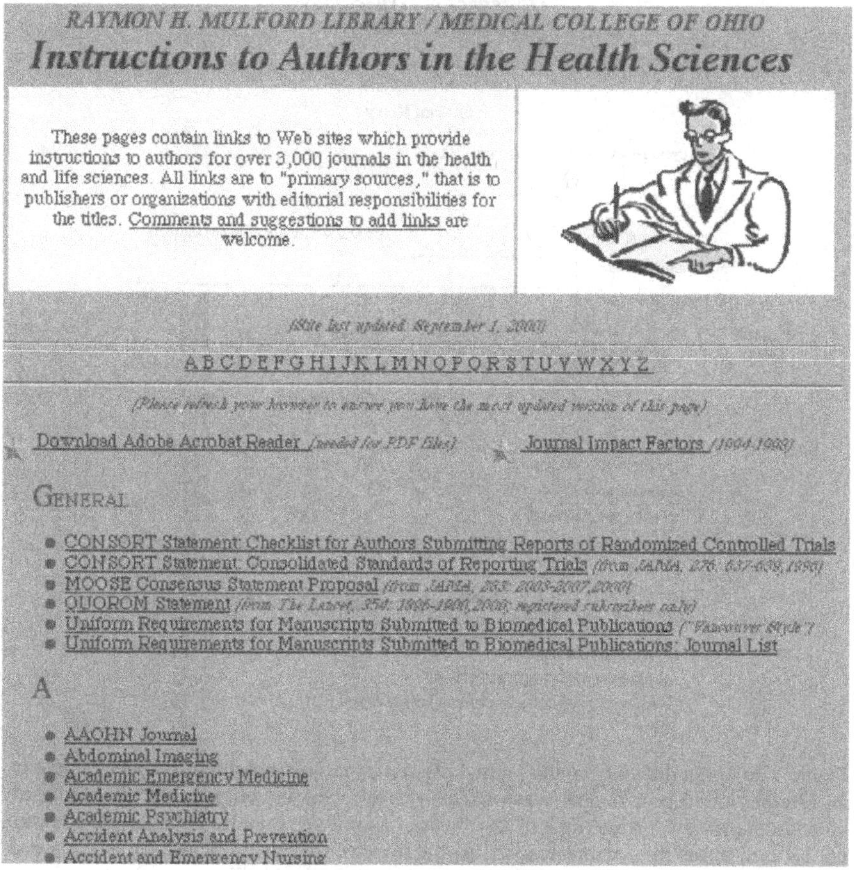

Figure 7.3. The Raymon H. Mulford Instructions to Authors site is a must for any author of a medically related work. (**http://www.mco.edu/lib/instr/libinsta.html**)

Peer Review

A number of medical journals now offer peer reviewers an opportunity to submit manuscript reviews over the Internet. While the format varies from journal to journal, most allow the reviewer's comments to the authors and editors to be either typed directly into a text box at the site or pasted from material created in a word processor. A "send" button on the page is clicked and the information sent to the editorial staff. In some cases, word processing files are directly sent either by e-mail or as FTP attachments. Some journals include a checklist or rating scale that completes the evaluation process (Fig. 7.4). Because of the nature of blinded peer review, when these systems are provided they are password protected and they can only be used for the submission of the review—somewhat like a very specialized electronic mail system. Unlike a standard

Obstetrics & Gynecology
Manuscript Review

Editorial Report

Submit your review to: ● *Los Angeles* (default)
                        ○ *Seattle*

Reviewer: _____

Reviewer Email: _____   (You will receive a copy at this address)

Manuscript Number: _____

First Author Name: _____

Please rate the manuscript by checking the appropriate box:

	best		average		worst
	1	2	3	4	5
Importance to this journal:	○	○	○	○	○
Adequacy of methods:	○	○	○	○	○
Results and interpretation:	○	○	○	○	○
Overall quality:	○	○	○	○	○

Recommendation

Accept in present form	○
Accept contingent upon minor revisions	○
Major revision needed; accept if appropriately revised	○
Reject	○

Figure 7.4. Again drawn from the journal *Obstetrics & Gynecology,* this is an example of an Internet-based peer review system. This site is accessible only with a password provided to the reviewer at the time of the review, can only be used for submission, and cannot be used to see the comments made by the reviewer or others. (Space for the required narrative comments is provided below the portion shown in this illustration.)

e-mail system, these pages send information to the editorial staff, but cannot retrieve, receive, or display information. This prevents anyone except the editors from seeing the results of the review. Even the reviewers themselves cannot see the information again once it has been sent. This is in keeping with the function of the Web page as simply a conduit, but it also protects the privacy of author and reviewer alike.

Manuscript Transfer and Editing

In some fields of science, most notably physics, journals have arisen that are completely electronic from Internet submission to paperless subscriptions. Most medical journals, however, are still paper based for the initial parts of the submission and review process. For papers that are close to final acceptance, some journals accept or require authors to provide a copy of their work in electronic form (most often on a magnetic disk). Most publishers who do this accept a variety of word-processing formats or text (ASCII) files. Whether your manuscript

Table 7.1. Guidelines for electronic submission of manuscripts

Be certain to include a printout of the version of the article that is submitted.
Put only the latest version of the manuscript on the disk or as an attachment.
Name the file clearly and be sensitive to naming conventions for various operating systems (e.g., IBM vs. Mac).
Label the disk with the format of the file and the file name or include the information in the body of the e-mail message.
Provide information about the hardware and software used to create the file.
Do not use a file compression program unless requested by the publisher. Use only programs that are available to, and compatible for, both users.

is to be submitted on a disk or as an attachment to an electronic mail, you must be careful to inform the recipient about the form and format used to store the information contained. Some general guidelines for electronic submissions are shown in Table 7.1.

Authors should consult the journal's instructions to authors for acceptable formats, conventions for naming files, number of (paper) copies to be submitted, and other details.

If you are going to submit a manuscript as a text file attachment to electronic mail, there are some additional considerations: In the body of the message be sure to include the same information contained in Table 7.1. You may know exactly what this is all about, but the person who opens the editor's overflowing electronic mailbox may not. Therefore, be sure to give information about the intent of the submission in addition to the formatting information. Some e-mail systems "encapsulate" attachments with specialized information placed before and after the file itself. This allows the e-mail system and the Internet to identify the type of file being sent, its length, format, and other characteristics. This encapsulation may take place at many points along the transmission route resulting in a file with electronic "garbage" at either end. Consequently, occasionally the receiving computer may not recognize a file as being in a format that it can interpret. This is most likely to happen when the sending and receiving computers are using different e-mail programs, browsers, or operating systems. To see if this will be a problem, send a short test file first to ensure that both parties can send, receive, and open the document correctly. It is easier to sort out the protocols at this stage than when sending a 2.1-megabit chapter (such as Chapter 5 of this book). If a problem persists, consider using a compression program to shrink and encode the file before transmission. These compression programs can often provide the needed protection to retain the integrity of the original file and may drastically reduce the time it takes to transmit the file. Do be sure that the receiving party has the required decompression software or that the file has been made self-extracting.

On-line Journals

The contents of many medical journals may be directly accessed using the Internet. Abstracts and other elements have traditionally been available through systems such as MedLine. Increasingly, the entire contents of journals are available through Internet access. For most journals, this is restricted to paid subscribers and may be limited to past issues. In some cases, the current issue is immediately available (Fig. 7.5). When this service is available, the tables of contents are hyperlinked to the articles themselves. The articles are generally presented, as they would be on the printed page, complete with tables, graphs, and illustrations. In many cases, the footnotes used for references are hyperlinked to either the citation in the paper's bibliography or to the original reference itself. Even if the entire contents of the journal are not openly accessible, many sites will offer the text of selected article. An example of this is the *JAMA* Web site offered by the American Medical Association (**jama.ama-assn.org**). Here selected articles of special interest are offered to the public in their full-text version. The special position of *JAMA* as a more public forum makes this public access both appropriate and logical. Other journals, such as *The Lancet* (**www.thelancet.com**), *The New England Journal of Medicine* (**www.nejm. com**), and the general journal *Science* (**www.sciencemag.org**), take a similar stance, making publicly accessible supplementary files and full-text versions for many of their major articles.

Access to printed journals can be obtained on-line through several intermediary Internet sites. An example of this type of service is BioMedNet.Com (**http://www.bmn.com**). BioMedNet.com offers registered users access to print journals, but in some cases there is a fee for downloading the articles that varies from $2.50 to $10.00. To access your subscription on line, you register the journal's name, your user's name, and a reader's code from the mailing label of the journal. Your print subscription is verified with the publisher and an access code sent to you to allow direct on line access.

OBSTETRICS& GYNECOL●GY

September 2000
Volume 96, Number 3

Previous issues

Jodi S. Dashe, Donald D. McIntire, Michael J. Lucas, and Kenneth J. Leveno	Effects of Symmetric and Asymmetric Fetal Growth on Pregnancy Outcomes
Lorenzo Guariglia and Paolo Rosati	Transvaginal Sonographic Detection of Embryonic-Fetal Abnormalities in Early Pregnancy
Andrew Elimian, Uma Verma, Debra Beneck, Rebecca Cipriano, Paul Visintainer, and Nergesh Tejani	Histologic Chorioamnionitis, Antenatal Steroids, and Perinatal Outcomes
Wolfgang Eppel, Christof Worda, Peter Frigo, Martin Ulm, Elisabeth Kucera, and Klaus Czerwenka	Human Papillomavirus in the Cervix and Placenta

Figure 7.5. Some medical journals provide Internet access to the contents of current issues. This example is again drawn from the journal *Obstetrics & Gynecology*.

MedLine and Literature Repositories

No physician or other health professional can escape the processes of education and training without becoming familiar with the various resources for finding information in the medical literature. In the electronic arena, the longest running of these resources is the National Library of Medicine's (NLM) MedLine system. Growing out of the printed indexes of the recent past, the electronic version offers speed, power, and the possibility of access from clinics, offices, libraries, and hotel rooms. MedLine serves 50,000 users a day and provides the results of over nine million searches per month. As a resource, MedLine is so important to the practice of medicine that we will devote a major portion of Chapter 8 to its effective use.

The Internet (and the sites available on it) makes it possible to access the body of medical literature using a number of search and navigation engines, the most familiar of which is the NLM's MedLine. MedLine is only one of more than 40 databases offered on-line by NLM. While MedLine is a service of the National Library of Medicine, over 100 licensees of NLM's databases (Ovid and others) provide either direct access or a specialized interface that acts as an intermediate agent. An example of an intermediary type of system is the NLM's own PubMed. PubMed is an experimental service of the National Center for Biotechnology Information (NCBI) at the National Library of Medicine. Established in 1988 as a national resource for molecular biology information, NCBI offers public databases, conducts research in computational biology, develops tools for analyzing genome data, and disseminates biomedical information through its Web site and other activities. PubMed was developed in conjunction with publishers of biomedical literature as a search tool for accessing literature citations and linking to their full-text versions at publishers' Web sites. PubMed searches the 10 million records (30,000+ added each month) in MedLine supplemented by pre-MedLine citations that do not yet have Medical Subject Headings (MeSH) index terms and by citations supplied electronically by publishers. Independent and commercial sites that link to MedLine or PubMed often allow seamless access to other literature databases such as GenBank, Genomes, ToxLine, and others. The National Center for Biomedical Information (**www.ncbi.nlm.nih.gov**) offers PubMed access as well as some of these specialized databases. Free links to MedLine and PubMed have now become common enough that there are even sites that offer lists of links (**www.docnet.org.uk/drfelix**).

Another access point is the Grateful Med site, also operated by the National Library of Medicine (Fig. 7.6). Like other portals, this site uses the search engine of PubMed, but offers access to a wider group of literature databases in medicine, biology, and other sciences. Queries carried out through the Grateful Med site gives results by searching in 14 other databases using NLM's MEDLARS system. The Grateful Med site also offers access to Loansome Doc, a service that allow you to obtain hard copies of medical references and other documents. There is a fee for this service, but for those without access to a traditional medical library (a "lonesome" doc), the service can more than pay for itself. Grateful Med also offers direct links to nearly 60,000 images at its Images from the History of Medicine.

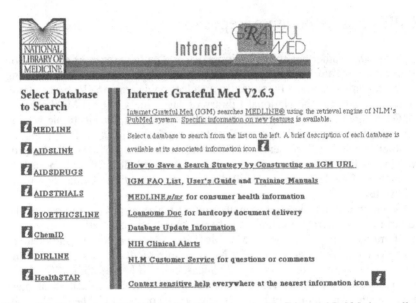

Figure 7.6. The Grateful Med Web site offers access to MedLine and PubMed as well as other biomedical, biologic, and scientific literature databases. (**igm.nlm.nih.gov**)

Textbooks and References

The Internet offers access to the content of traditional texts in two ways: access to publishers and booksellers offering print versions, and direct access to the electronic form of the printed text. Many publishers have Web pages that allow the visitor to search the list of books available directly from the publisher, read descriptions or reviews, and place orders on-line (Fig. 7.7). Most of these sites have lists that are organized by specialty or topic. Titles may also be found through site search engines that find volumes by title, topic, or author. Many of the larger Internet bookstores, such as Amazon.com or Barnes and Noble (**www.bn.com**), have sections that deal with medical topics or search engines that will help find a particular title. While larger dealers will often carry the textbooks and references used by the major specialties, very technical works or those with a smaller audience may not be stocked.

The second manner of textbook access is through a Web connection to the electronic form of the content. This usually requires the payment of a renewable or continuing subscription fee and the use of a user name and password. The Internet now offers over 33 different titles through three different Web-based products: Scientific American Medicine Online, Harrison's Online, and Stat!Ref. These products allow comprehensive searching across titles and searching that can be narrowly focused to individual chapters or pages. Illustrations, graphics, and charts are also supported and searchable.

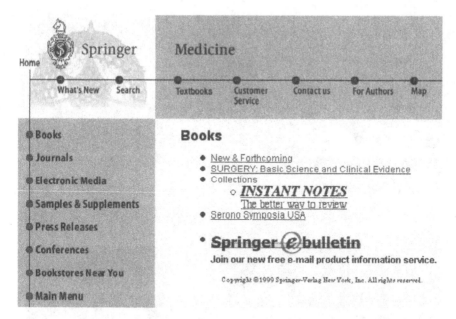

Figure 7.7. The Web site of Springer-Verlag is typical of that offered by medical publishers. At this site, the visitor can view descriptions of texts and place orders directly. (**http://www.springer-ny.com**)

One of the most popular sites of this type is the Harrison's Online offering *Harrison's Textbook of Medicine* (Fig. 7.8). For an annual subscription fee of $89 (at the time of this writing) the user can search the entire contents of the textbook. Included are links to update and clinical trial articles, PreTests, and a list of sites related to the chapter. Hyperlinks allow you to click on the author's last name to learn about his or her professional affiliation, other articles contributed to Harrison's Online, and publications listed in MedLine. The on-line versions of these textbooks are always the most current, with updated material that is added more quickly and more frequently than would be possible with printed material. Frequently included are extra graphs, tables, illustrations, and sound or video clips that enhance the content and would not be possible in any other media. The navigation tools familiar to users of print medium are all available, including table of contents and index. In addition, specialized forms of the table of contents, site maps, links to related information, and other navigation tools make access more efficient.

Some publicly accessible databases are moving to make selected texts available on-line. In collaboration with book publishers, NCBI is adapting texts for the Web and linking them to PubMed. The idea is to provide background information to PubMed, so that users can explore unfamiliar concepts found in PubMed search results. On any PubMed abstract page there is a "Books" button that takes the user to a facsimile of the abstract, in which some phrases are hypertext links. These phrases correspond to terms that are also found in the books available at NCBI. Clicking on a hypertext link takes the reader to a list of book

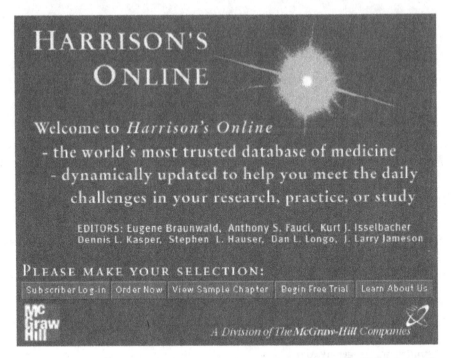

Figure 7.8. McGraw-Hill publishing makes their *Harrison's Textbook of Medicine* available to subscribers to the service. (**www.harrisonsonline.com**)

pages in which the phrase is found. When readers have accessed the page, they can navigate around other pages within that section of the book to research their topic further. Each unit stands alone and includes the corresponding figures, tables, and reference citations, which are linked where possible back to PubMed abstracts. The first book to be adapted and posted, *Biology of the Cell*, 3rd ed., by Bruce Alberts, Dennis Bray, Julian Lewis, Martin Raff, Keith Roberts, and James D. Watson, published by Garland Publishing, Inc., is now available. Rather than mirroring the textbook in print (i.e., treating the book as a whole, to be read sequentially from the first page to the last), the book is divided into units of content based on the organization of chapters, sections, subsections, etc., within the book. The entry point for a user is a page linked appropriately to a relevant PubMed abstract.

One advantage that this emerging structure conveys is the ability to link the on-line textbook to the resources of the MedLine database. References cited in the book are linked to their PubMed abstracts by using the Citation Matcher. This gives the reader a starting point to explore further the literature using PubMed's "Related Articles" function. Because books usually carry established knowledge, the references cited within them are often several years old; using Related Articles, a reader can move forward in time to find similar, more recent articles.

While there is little doubt that electronic textbooks offer enhanced capabilities and value, there are obvious drawbacks. Aside from the continuing cost of subscription is the issue of access. With a printed text, I can carry the information almost anywhere without regard to power or Internet connections. What I save in bulk I pay for in location restrictions. Unless you are a total propeller head or geek, it is not likely that you will read the electronic version of a text in the bathroom or on the beach, but you could do so with a printed version. An intermediate option is the CD-ROM form of many texts. These are lighter, smaller, and easier to pack, but still require a computer or electronic book. Interestingly, at a 2000 meeting of the American Psychological Association, a study was presented that indicated that on-line readers (or those of electronic books) found the authors less credible and arguments less persuasive than for printed text. Printed text was seen to be more interesting and comprehensible. Certainly, personal preference and taste are the ultimate arbiters.

Special Text Resources

The Internet offers a number of resources to assist in the craft of writing. If you need a dictionary, even in a foreign language, you can consult one on-line. An example of such a site is **www.yourdictionary.com**. This site combines both standard dictionary functions and those of a thesaurus. It piques a word lover's interest with a word of the day (Fig. 7.9), specialized dictionaries, guides to the origins of words, pronunciation, acronyms, synonyms, homophones, lexicography, and more. Even if you only occasionally compose e-mail, this site can help make your text richer. (Wandering the site in view of others can also improve your social status in some circles, but may hurt your dating chances if you are single.)

Today's Word:

Rubefacient (Adjective)

Pronunciation: [ru-bê-'fey-shênt]

Definition 1: Causing redness (usually in the skin); an agent that causes redness (Noun).

Usage 1: The term is usually used in the medical sense, but why stop there

Suggested usage: Certain allergens are rubefacient but so is an embarrassing remark if it results in blushing. "Rubefacient language" or "remark" is a nice euphemism for "profanity" or anything spoken out of place. "The document was a rubefacient for all who worked on it."

Etymology: Latin rubefacere "to make red", itself from rubeus "reddish" + facere "to make". Rubeus is from PIE reudh-, the origin of ruby, red, robust, corroborate, rambunctious, ruddy, rust, and rouge. From facere (PPart fact-us) fact, faction, factor, fashion, feasible, feat, and feature are derived.

—Dr. Language, yourDictionary.com

Figure 7.9. The word of the day is a feature of YourDictionalry.com. (**http://www. yourdictionary.com**)

One last group of Internet assets that warrant special mention are the translation tools that allow the user to move information from one language to another. This ranges from Internet dictionaries to sites that will perform the translation of typed text directly. This translation process, while helpful, is not without its limitations (Table 7.2). The capabilities that these sites provide are helpful for interpreting foreign language abstracts or short documents, but should not be used for the development of final text, patient-related materials, or foreign submissions—nothing takes the place of a talented translator or native speaker.

Table 7.2 Translation of a section of text from above to and from French by Transparent Language at FreeTranslation.com (**www.freetranslation.com**)

Original text	French translation	Translation back
This translation process, while helpful, is not without its limitations. The capabilities that these sites provide are helpful for interpreting foreign language abstracts or short documents, but should not be used for the development of final text, patient-related materials, or foreign submissions—nothing takes the place of a talented translator or native speaker.	Ce procédé de traduction, pendant que serviable, n'est pas sans ses limitations. Les capacités que ces sites fournissent sont serviables pour interpréter les résumés de langue étrangers ou les documents courts, mais ne devrait pas être utilisé pour le développement de texte final, le malade matériels relatés ou submissions étranger—rien ne prend l'endroit d'un traducteur doué ou un haut-parleur natal.	This translation procedure, while serviable, is not without its limitations. The capacities that these sites furnish are serviable to interpret the foreigners language or the courts documents, but should not be used for the development final text, sick equipment related or submissions foreigner—nothing does not take the place of a gifted translator or a natal high-speaker.

8
Finding Medical Information

Medical Information Searches

Finding medical and medically related information on the Internet is not dramatically different from finding any other information. The same techniques that we discussed in Chapter 3 can be broadly applied to medical topics. However, several significant differences must be kept in mind to make your medically related searching easier and more productive.

Search Engines and Tools

While you can use the same search engines outlined earlier to perform medically related searches, their efficiency is often disappointing. A search for "stroke" is more likely to turn up Web sites that offer to help with your golf game than to turn up sites that sort out your neurologic findings. To get around this problem, you must use either smarter search strategies or different tools.

If you use a standard Internet search engine for a medical topic, you will have greater success finding sites of help if you give the search engine guidance about your needs. If you want to locate a site the gives you the latest research on anticoagulant use in acute stroke, take advantage of Boolean search terms to restrict your investigation. Using a strategy such as "stroke AND therapy" or "stroke AND anticoagulants" will dramatically reduce the number of sites unrelated to your interest. This works well if you have a well-defined topic that can be concisely delimited. If you are unsure, use more nonspecific modifiers such as "AND medicine," "AND brain," or a similar general term. The list of sites returned may suggest other modifiers or other search techniques. Some search engines include buttons or links associated with their results pages that will take you directly to related sites or searches.

Often a more efficient strategy for finding medical information is to use sites or resources that are specifically designed for the medical information. These may include obvious sites such as the National Library of Medicine's MedLine or PubMed (discussed below) or less apparent sources of search and referral. Many professional organizations or disease-specific sites will have either internal search engines or links to sites that are related or germane to the purpose of the parent organization or site. An example of this type of internal search is the search options made available to members of the American College of Obstetricians and Gynecologists (Fig. 8.1). At this members-only section of the site, users can enter complex search terms to retrieve information from College publications or the journal *Obstetrics & Gynecology*.

Not all sources of specialized medical links are offered by official organizations. Smaller organizations, corporations, or even individuals may maintain useful links as well. Corporate sites that specialize in medical information and medical links, such as Medical Matrix, have been illustrated earlier. In addition to these sites, there are some notable individual sites as well. As we have

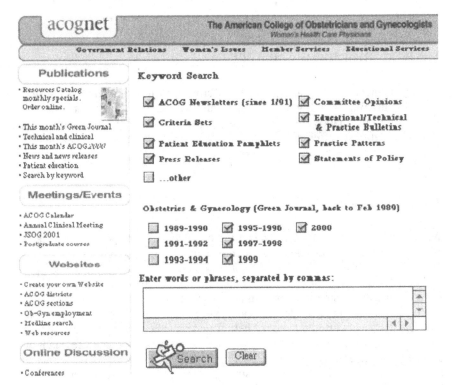

Figure 8.1. Many professional organizations offer their members specialized search tools to locate information of interest. This members-only example is from the American College of Obstetricians and Gynecologists.

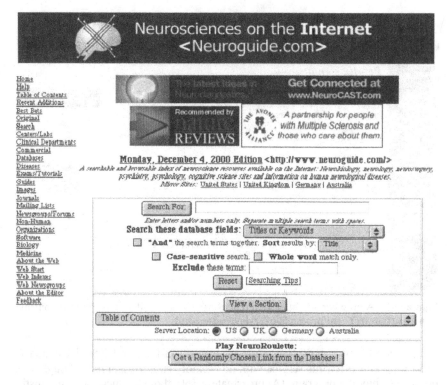

Figure 8.2. Web pages maintained by interested (and dedicated) individuals can be a useful source of, or links to, medical information. (**www.neuroguide.com**)

observed, some care should be exercised in evaluating the reliability of less official sites; this said, some outstanding examples of useful sites do exist. An example is the Neuroguide site (Fig. 8.2). This site is edited and maintained by Neil A. Busis, M.D., a neurologist at the University of Pittsburgh. The site offers several ways for users to search for neuroscientific information, including a roulette option that takes users to a random site of possible interest.

Filters

A brief (no pun intended) discussion of pornography, and content filters is in order because they can significantly affect searches for medical information. Many physicians use their home computers for medical information purposes. If they have children, or merely prefer to avoid inadvertent display of materials that they find objectionable, they may use Internet filter programs such as Net Nanny (for IBM computers), CyberPatrol (IBM & Mac, Fig. 8.3), or others. With these programs, the user has the ability to decide which Web sites are appropriate and which are not. These programs use pre-prepared lists of potentially objectionable sites and the user can add or modify this for their own purposes. Other features include complete activity logs, choice of actions if a violation

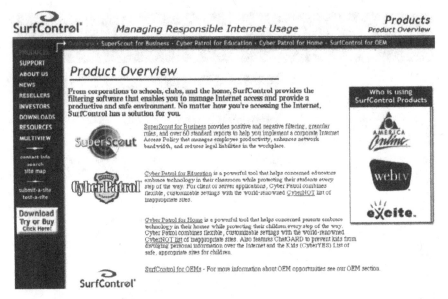

Figure 8.3. A number of Internet content filters is available from SurfControl. (**www.surfcontrol.com/products/overview/index.html**)

occurs, control over how long children can be on-line, and free list updates. Most programs offer this service with no monthly subscription fees, though you do have to buy the program. (Approximately $50, though educational and institutional discounts are available.)

These Internet filters vary in their flexibility and efficiency in achieving their task as policemen. In general, the more efficient the system is in blocking materials or thwarting inquisitive teenagers, the more inflexible and complex the program and the more difficult it is to customize it to your own needs. When Internet filters are used, they may make it impossible to reach medically related sites for homework or professional purposes. Sites that can be blocked vary from the American Society of Breast Surgery to Beaver College, a Presbyterian school founded in 1853 and located in Glenside, PA. (The school recently changed its name for this very reason.) This can even extend to sites with less inflammatory names, such as the American Cancer Society, when the site's content contains words on the forbidden list. The result is that if you are going to search for medically related information, you should plan on disabling the filter program (a sometimes difficult option) or not using one to begin with.

MedLine and PubMed

The importance and utility of the National Library of Medicine's (NLM) databases MedLine and PubMed make a brief discussion of their use and of the search strategies used within these sites worthwhile. As we have discussed above, without an efficient search strategy, the wealth of information contained at these sites is inaccessible and may as well not exist at all.

The NLM uses a classification scheme for all of the articles that it indexes. This consists of the basic information about the article such as authors, title, journal, volume, issue, pages, language, type of subjects (human or animal), etc. In addition to this, each article is assigned to a Medical Subject Heading (MeSH). This heading system consists of a controlled vocabulary of hierarchical terms. This nesting of terms allows subjects and topics to be grouped together in logical ways, streamlining searches and ensuring more complete recovery of relevant items. The search engines that MedLine and PubMed employ use these terms as both heading and text words as appropriate. In addition, the search engine "explodes" parent terms to include more specific child (sub) terms in the search. For example, if the user enters "Filovirus," the system will search on "Filovirus" and add in its more specific subterms, "Ebola virus" and "Marburg virus." In addition, the software has the ability to map invalid requests to valid MeSH headings. For example, "Megacolon/congenital" maps to "Hirschsprung disease."

The search system has a "just do it" system that attempts to correct for user errors. In this aspect of the system, there are nearly 5,000 mappings for associated expressions (e.g., "Plasma Separators" maps to "Plasma AND Cell Separation/Instrumentation") and hundreds of mappings for relatively unambiguous synonyms of search qualifiers (e.g., "adverse reaction," "side effects," and "undesirable effects" all map to "adverse effects"). The search system also uses a unified language system. NLM's Unified Medical Language System Metathesaurus acts as an electronic Rosetta stone with the 1998 version containing 1,052,000 names for 476,000 concepts in more than 40 biomedical vocabularies, thesauri, and classifications. (The computer also contains French, German, Spanish, Portuguese, and transliterated Russian translations of MeSH system.) These functions increase the effectiveness of the search engine while keeping the number of MeSH headings logical and manageable.

Because the PubMed interface offers the most powerful tools for interpreting search requests, we will look specifically at using the PubMed system. To take advantage of the computing power offered, you begin by entering the terms you wish to search for in the blank (query box) on the main screen for the site (Fig. 8.4). You can enter one or more search terms, or click Preview/Index for advanced searching options. You may enter one or more terms (e.g., vitamin c common cold) in the query box, and PubMed automatically combines (ANDs) significant terms together using the automatic term mapping discussed earlier. The terms are searched in the various fields of the citation. Once you click Go, PubMed will display your search results while a separate "Details" box can display your search terms as you entered them. The black bar at the top of the display contains links to PubMed and the other NCBI resources. The Features bar directly beneath the query box provides access to additional search options. Both the PubMed query box and Features bar remain available from every screen, allowing a new search to start without returning to the home (first) page.

Searches may (and often should) include Boolean or logical operators. (If your search includes the Boolean operators AND, OR, NOT, they must be in upper case.) The PubMed search engine processes the Boolean connectors in a

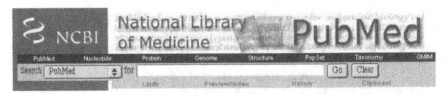

Figure 8.4. Search terms are entered into the blank at the PubMed opening screen. (**www.ncbi.nlm.nih.gov/entrez/query.fcgi**)

left-to-right sequence. Consequently, the following search statements will not return the same information:

> Common cold AND vitamin C OR Zinc
> Common cold OR vitamin C AND Zinc

In the first statement, the citations for the common cold will be compared with those for vitamin C and those with references to both will be combined with citations referring to zinc (in any way). In the second search, citations will be gathered that refer to either the common cold or vitamin C and these will be grouped together. This group will then be compared to a list of citations for zinc, and only those in both groups will be returned. This is a seemingly subtle, but very important difference.

You can change the order that PubMed processes a search statement by enclosing individual concepts in parentheses. The terms inside the set of parentheses will be processed as a unit and then incorporated into the overall strategy, e.g., common cold AND (vitamin c OR zinc). If PubMed finds a phrase within a search strategy string that uses unqualified terms (those that are not part of the MeSH system), it will automatically search the terms as a phrase rather than simply combining the individual words. For example, if you enter "air bladder fistula" in the PubMed search box, PubMed will search "air bladder" as a phrase. If you do not want this automatic phrase parsing, your should enter each term separated by AND, e.g., air AND bladder AND fistula. If you are uncertain, click on Details to see how your search strategy was implemented (Fig. 8.5). (If you place a tag qualifier, discussed below, it should follow the relevant term and precede the Boolean operator.)

Once you have entered your search items and clicked on Go, PubMed returns the results of your inquiry in a results box (Fig. 8.6). PubMed search results are displayed with the most recent listed first. At the top of the display are buttons that allow you to display additional information about any citations that you indicate by clicking on the check box to the left of the entry. These display options include the ability to show the brief, abstract, full citation, or to obtain links to other databases. Checked items may be saved, downloaded as a text file to your computer, or ordered in printed form (for a fee). Below these buttons, options for determining which of the retrieved citations are displayed are offered. These include the number of citations per "page" and the starting point or page to be displayed. Each citation is hyperlinked to the abstract of the paper and links to related articles (Fig. 8.7). This display carries a link to the publisher's Web site and related books or articles when appropriate. Again, a check

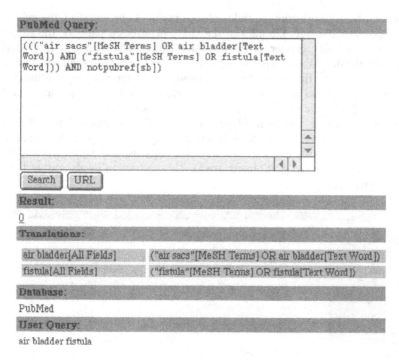

Figure 8.5. The PubMed "Details" display tells users how their search was executed. Changes in the search may be entered here or in the Limits section.

box is supplied so that you can flag the citation so that it can be saved, added to you clipboard, or placed in your "cubby[4]" for recall later.

You can modify your current search by adding or eliminating terms in the query box, in Details (Fig. 8.8), or by supplying limits on the search strategy. The PubMed Details box shows the actual search strategy and syntax used to run the search. Directly beneath this box is displayed the result number. This tells the number of citations returned and is hyperlinked to displays of the matches for the current search. The Translations area details how each term was translated using PubMed's search rules and syntax, and the User Query area shows the search terms as you entered them in the query box. To edit the search strategy in the query box, click in the box to add or delete terms and then click Search. To return to the current search results screen, you click this link or use the "Back" function of your Web browser.

Clicking on the Limits link, located just below the window where search terms were entered, places limits on the search. Once you click on this link, a new dialog screen appears to assist with refining your search. Here you supply limits that act as inclusion or exclusion criteria that the search engine uses so that the citations returned more closely fit your needs. In other words, limits remove unneeded or unwanted documents. The most commonly used

---

[4] Just like in kindergarten, a cubby is a place where you can keep search strategies, that may be updated at any time. In order for you to use this feature your Web browser must be set to accept cookies.

limits are those that restrict the fields of information to be searched, the publication type, the language, the ages of the study or affected patients, the subject (human vs. animal), gender, or the date publication. These options vary somewhat with the database in use. The options available in the PubMed database for each of these limit fields are shown in Table 8.1. When you apply limits to a search, they apply to the search in general and not to the specific elements. If you apply limits, the check box next to limits will be marked and a listing of your limit selections will be displayed. To turn off the existing limits, click on the check box to remove the check before running your next search. To restrict citations to those with abstracts use the value "hasabstract" within your search terms (e.g., menopause AND hasabstract). This restriction needs neither limits nor tag qualifiers.

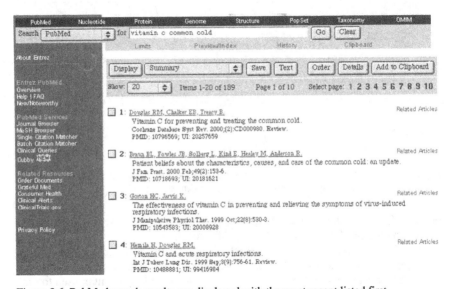

Figure 8.6. PubMed search results are displayed with the most recent listed first.

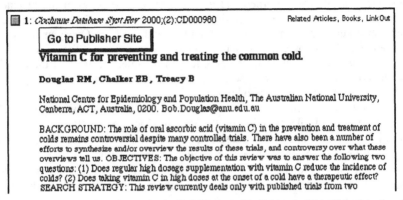

Figure 8.7. Each citation shown in the PubMed results display is hyperlinked to the abstract of the article (when available). When appropriate, a link to the publisher's Web site and related books or articles is also provided.

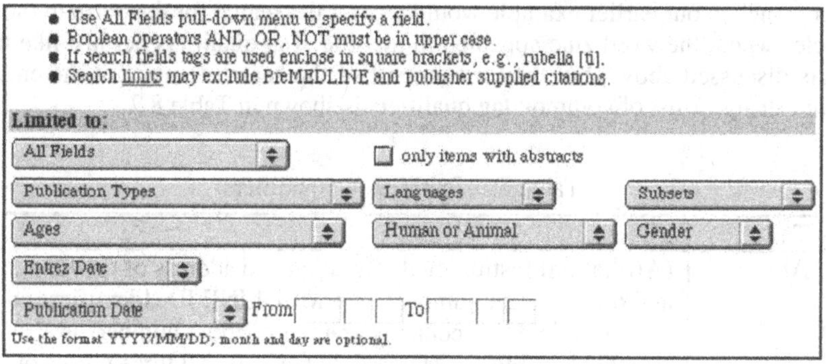

- Use All Fields pull-down menu to specify a field.
- Boolean operators AND, OR, NOT must be in upper case.
- If search fields tags are used enclose in square brackets, e.g., rubella [ti].
- Search limits may exclude PreMEDLINE and publisher supplied citations.

Limited to:

All Fields ⬍	☐ only items with abstracts
Publication Types ⬍	Languages ⬍	Subsets ⬍
Ages ⬍	Human or Animal ⬍	Gender ⬍
Entrez Date ⬍
Publication Date ⬍	From [ ] [ ] To [ ] [ ] [ ]

Use the format YYYY/MM/DD; month and day are optional.

Figure 8.8. The PubMed Limits screen allows you to place restrictions on the search for the terms entered on the primary search screen.

Table 8.1. Limit options for the PubMed database

Limit type	Options
Fields	Affiliation, all fields, author name, EC/RN number, entrez date, filter, issue, journal name, language, MeSH date, MeSH major topic, MeSH terms, page number, publication date, publication type, secondary source ID, subheading, substance name, text word, title word, title/abstract word, UID, volume
Publication type	Clinical trial, editorial, letter, meta-analysis, practice guideline, randomized clinical trial, review
Language	English, French, German, Italian, Japanese, Russian, Spanish
Subsets	AIDS, AIM, Dental, MedLine, Nursing, PreMedline, Publishers, PubRef, Toxicology
Ages	All infant: birth–23 months; all child: 0–18 years; all adult: 19+ years; newborn: birth–1 month; infant: 1–23 months; preschool child: 2–5 years; child: 6–12 years; adolescent: 13-18 years; adult: 19–44 years; middle aged: 45–64 years; aged: 65+ years; 80 and over: 80+ years
Human or animal	Human, animal
Gender	Female, male
Entrez date	30 days, 60 days, 90 days, 108 days, 1 year, 2 years, 5 years, 10 years
Publication date	A date range in the format YYYY/MM/DD; month and day are optional

Another way of applying limits to a search is to use a tag qualifier. These are codes of two or more letters placed inside square brackets that tell the search engine to restrict the search in some manner. For example, placing the code [TI] after "zinc" in our earlier example would restrict the search for that term to those articles where the word zinc appeared in the title. Tag qualifiers act just like the limits discussed above, but they act on part of the search terms, not the entire search string. A list of common tag qualifiers is shown in Table 8.2

Table 8.2. PubMed tag qualifiers

Tag	Effect
AD	(Affiliation) Institutional affiliation and address of the first author, and grant numbers. The MEDLINE ID (Identification Number) field that contains grant or contract numbers is also searchable using the search field tag [ad]. All three pieces of the ID field (actual number, grant acronym, and institute mnemonic) are each individually searchable.
ALL	(All Fields) Includes all searchable PubMed fields. However, only terms where there is no match found in one of the Translation tables or Indexes via the Automatic Term Mapping process will be searched in All Fields.
AU	(Author) Searches within the Author field for the specified name. The format to search for an author name is: last name followed by a space and up to the first two initials followed by a space and a suffix abbreviation, if applicable, all without periods or a comma after the last name (e.g., smith rp or smith se jr). Initials and suffixes may be omitted when searching the author field.
DP	(Publication Date) The date that the article was published. Dates or date ranges must be searched using the format YYYY/MM/DD [dp]. The month and day are optional (e.g., 1998 [dp] or 1998/03 [dp]). To enter a date range, insert a colon between each date.
EDAT	(Entrez Date) Date the citation was added to the PubMed database. The Entrez Date is set to the Publication Date on citations before September 1997 when this field was first added to PubMed.
IP	(Journal issue) The number of the journal issue in which the article is published.
LA	(Language) The language in which the article was published. Note that many non-English articles have English-language abstracts. You can either enter the language or enter just the first three characters of most languages, e.g., chi [la] retrieves the same as chinese [la]. The most notable exception is jpn [la] for Japanese.
MH	(MeSH heading) This restricts the search to the NLM's Medical Subject Headings controlled vocabulary of biomedical terms.
PG	(Page Number) Enter only the first page number for the article. The citation will display the full pagination of the article but this field is searchable using only the first page number.

Table 8.2. PubMed tag qualifiers

Tag	Effect
PS	(Personal Name as Subject) Use this search field tag to limit retrieval to where the name is the subject of the article, e.g., varmus h [ps]. The search rules for Author [au] apply to this field.
PT	(Publication Type) Describes the type of material the article represents (e.g., Review, Clinical Trial, Retracted Publication, Letter).
SB	(Subset) The PubMed database is a combination of several NLM databases, MEDLINE, PreMEDLINE, and Health-STAR journal citations. This tag qualifier allows you to search only a part of the overall database.
SH	(Subheading) Subheadings are used with MeSH terms to help describe more completely a particular aspect of a subject. Subheadings automatically include the more specific sub-heading terms under the term in a search. To turn off this automatic feature, use the search syntax [sh:noexp], e.g., therapy [sh:noexp]. You can also enter the MEDLINE two-letter subheading abbreviations rather than spelling out the subheading, e.g., dh [sh] = diet therapy [sh].
SN	(Substance Name) The name of a chemical discussed in the article.
TA	(Journal title) This restriction will search the journal title ab-breviation, full journal name, or ISSN number. The Journal Browser is also available from the PubMed home page side-bar to look up the full name, abbreviation, and ISSN number of a journal. If a journal name contains parentheses or brack-ets, enter the name without the parentheses or brackets.
TI	(Title Word) Searches only for words and numbers included in the title of a citation.
TIAB	(Title/Abstract Words) Words and numbers included in the title and abstract of a citation.
TW	(Text Word) This is a very powerful tag to use when you can't seem to find the article you know is there somewhere. When this tag is used, the search includes all words and num-bers in the title and abstract, and MeSH terms, subheadings, chemical substance names, personal name as subject, and MEDLINE Secondary Source (SI) field.
VI	(Volume) The number of the journal volume in which an arti-cle is published.

If no match is found for your search, PubMed breaks apart the phrase and re-peats the automatic term mapping process until a match is found. If there is still no match, the individual terms will be combined (ANDed) together and searched in All Fields. When these automatic processes fail, there are several options that can still result in finding a citation. One trick is to use is truncation. Truncation allows you to find all of the terms that begin with the text string you specify. To use truncation, you place an asterisk at the end of the text string to be used for the search. The search will then return all terms that begin with that word; for instance bacter* will find all terms that begin with the letters bacter, e.g., bacteria, bacterium, bacteriophage, etc. PubMed searches are limited to the first 150 variations of a truncated term. If a truncated term produces more than 150 variations, PubMed displays a warning message. When this happens, expand the length of the text string (root word) that precedes the asterisk. Be aware that phrases that include a space in a word after the asterisk will not be included; for example, infection* includes infections, but not infection control. The use of truncation also turns off automatic term mapping and the automatic explosion of a MeSH term. For example, heart attack* will not map to the MeSH term Myocardial Infarction or include any of the more specific terms, e.g., Myocardial Stunning; Shock, Cardiogenic.

Another technique that can help to focus your search is phrase searching. PubMed consults a phrase index and groups terms into logical phrases. For example, if you enter poison ivy, PubMed recognizes this as a phrase and searches it as one search term. However, not all phrases are recognized as such and as a result, PubMed may fail to find a phrase that is essential to a search. For instance, if you enter single cell, it is not in the Phrase List, and PubMed will try to search for "single" and "cell" separately (as an AND search). To force PubMed to search for a specific phrase enter double quotes (" ") around the phrase, e.g., "single cell" (PubMed does not actually perform adjacency searching, but uses a list of recognized phrases against which search terms are matched). If your search phrase is not on the list of recognized phrases, then the double quotes are ignored and the phrase is processed using automatic term mapping. Consequently, your phrase may actually appear in the citation and abstract data, yet not be on the phrase list. To avoid this, add the tag qualifier (TW) to force the search process to directly match the phrase to the text of the citation. You should be aware that when you enclose a phrase in double quotes, PubMed will not perform its usual automatic term mapping. For example, "health planning" will include citations that are indexed to the MeSH term Health Planning, but will not include the more specific terms such as Health Care Rationing, Health Care Reform, Health Plan Implementation, and so on, that are included with the automatic MeSH mapping.

Sometimes it can be very helpful to save a search strategy for reuse later. To do this, click on the Details button in the results window. From the Details window, click on the URL button. When you click on the URL button, PubMed returns a URL that contains the search strategy information embedded within it. Use your browser to bookmark the URL for future use. Once you use your browser's bookmark function, you can edit the title, location, or other attributes of the bookmark to help you identify this URL for future use. To use the search again, simply click on the entry in your bookmark file, and the browser will pass on the required information to PubMed. Searches that were created using a search statement number in History, e.g., (#1 or #2 AND menopause [TW]), should not be saved using the URL feature since search statements represented by these numbers are lost when History is deleted. You may also save your search strategies using the Cubby function.

You should be aware that to perform some of its functions, PubMed uses cookies. Cookies allow PubMed to provide more interactive features such as Preview/Index, Clipboard, History, and the Cubby. Like other cookies, cookies placed by PubMed are removed from your computer after a set time. Therefore, you should set your browser either to allow cookies or to ask you before granting the placement of cookies. If your browser is set to deny all cookies, these functions will not work.

For those who wish to explore the PubMed and MedLine systems in greater depth, the NLM offers one- and two-day courses. Training materials for PubMed and Internet Grateful Med that correspond with the NLM's National Online Training Center training courses are available for downloading in PDF (portable document format) and WordPerfect 6.1 or higher formats (**www.nlm.nih.gov/ pubs/web_based.html**). The manuals have been broken down into sections so you can choose the areas of interest to you. PDF formats are best viewed with Adobe Acrobat Reader 4.0 or higher.

9
Continuing Medical Education

With links to information available at any time of day, to and from virtually any location on earth (with an Internet connection), it is apparent that the Internet can be, and is, a powerful tool for educational use. Whether used to support traditional self-prompted learning, such as reading, or the delivery of new learning opportunities, such as interactive multimedia, the Internet is playing a role. A recent search of the Internet for the terms "physician education" returned 521,207 possible matches. Internet-based continuing education is generally of low or no cost. It requires less time and no travel, while providing educational opportunities that are often enhanced by the incorporation of multimedia and the ability to continuously edit and refine the material offered.

Direct Education

Computer-aided instruction (CAI) for health professionals is gaining in popularity, based in great measure on the wide availability of simple, inexpensive Internet and computer tools. The first medical CAI systems were stand-alone show-case projects developed by and for academic centers. They were usually large, expensive, and limited in scope. Haken and associates at the University of Michigan used an intranet conferencing system that became an integral part of their student clerkship in obstetrics and gynecology. Using personal computers and terminals connected to the university mainframe computer by a local network, students could discuss selected topics with various faculty members, including the chairman. These teaching systems have gone as far as the use of virtual reality to facilitate training in surgical fields. Studies indicate that computer-based education compares favorably with traditional methods.

As with patient education systems, these programs are most effective when the computers are supported by audiovisual devices. Pictures and diagrams are especially important for the most common continuing medical education (CME) subjects. With a computer-video combination, any one of the more than 50,000 graphic images stored on a videodisk, DVD, or CD-ROM can be selected and displayed on the screen in a fraction of a second. The same video library used for CAI can also serve as an encyclopedic reference source in a physician's office. Unfortunately, the expense of producing videodisks limits the widespread use of this technology, but this has not been a factor for DVD- or CD-ROM-based systems. More and more of this technology is being ported to the Internet, which allows access to a constantly updated body of information supplied from a mainframe server.

A growing number of Internet sites offer direct continuing education opportunities. These range from the large general medical sites such as Medscape (Fig. 9.1) to small commercial ventures, from large universities to specialty groups. Medscape offers a selection of free, continuously updated continuing education activities for physicians, registered nurses, pharmacists, and other health professionals. All activities marked "CME" have been planned and implemented in accordance with the Essential Areas and Policies of the Accreditation Council for Continuing Medical Education (ACCME), and have been produced in collaboration with ACCME-accredited CME providers. The site offers on-line certificates of participation for most of the modules, and these are made available to users after they have completed a multiple choice test and course evaluation, both of which are submitted on-line. The site requires logging on, but membership and registration are free.

An interesting hybrid site is the Healthcare Learning and Information Exchange (HELIX) site supported by GlaxoWellcome (Fig. 9.2). This site offers

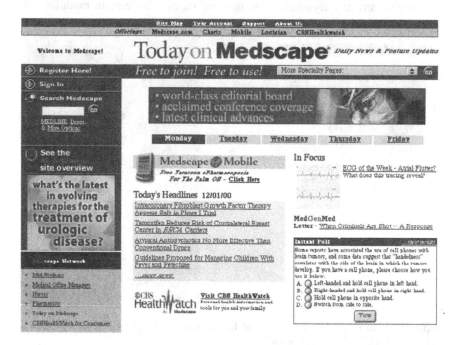

Figure 9.1. Medscape offers specialty specific introductory pages and continuing medical education in 19 specialty areas. (**www.medscape.com**)

continuing education in medicine, nursing, and pharmacy. In addition to on-line educational modules, the site offers information about scheduled lectures, teleconferences, and home study. Users select the appropriate category from a list provided on screen and proceed to the education area of their choice. Once you read the material, you complete an on-line posttest and submit it for grading. A passing grade results in granting of the desired credit. You do have to register, and the certificate is not available instantly online, but otherwise the system is similar to other on-line CME sites. Some physician education modules do require a fee, but these are reasonable compared to the cost of attending a conference.

An example of a for-profit continuing education site is CME Web (Fig. 9.3). This site offers a large variety of CME courses in a number of areas. These generally cost about $15 per credit hour, but the site offers the option of buying "in bulk" by paying a flat fee of $300 for a total of 60 credit hours. Registration does require the submission of a credit card number. In addition to the continuing education courses, a link provides a list of state by state continuing education requirements that can be useful if you are moving or are unsure of the current regulations that pertain to you. A total of almost 900 education modules are offered in 21 fields of medicine, with individual specialty offerings ranging from 3 to 165. Accreditation is through American Health Consultants, but some of the individual modules offer credit through specialty organizations such as the American Academy of Pediatrics, the American Academy of Family Physicians, the American College of Emergency Physicians, and The American College of Obstetricians and Gynecologists. In some cases, only certain modules are

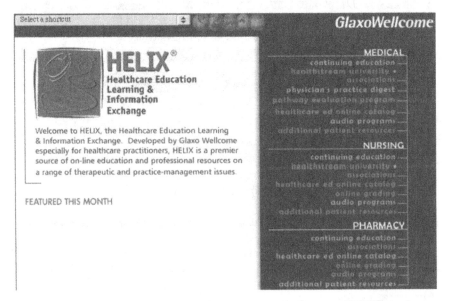

Figure 9.2. The Healthcare Learning and Information Exchange or HELIX site is supported by GlaxoWellcome (**www.helix.com**)

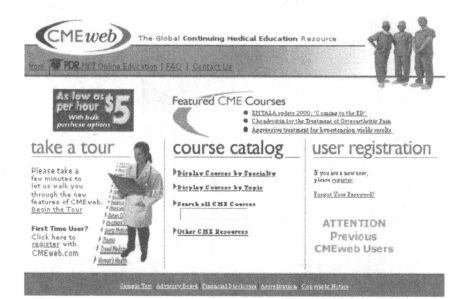

Figure 9.3. The CMEWeb site claims to be "the global continuing education resource." (**www.cmeweb.com**)

approved by these specialty bodies, and to obtain specialty credit you may have to submit the documentation directly to the organization.

Universities frequently offer educational opportunities that range from undergraduate course work to postgraduate continuing education. An example is the one offered by the University of Washington (Fig. 9.4). Informal education is available, though most modules require registration and the payment of a fee. The fee provides an inexpensive license that last for one year. Once you have your password, you can obtain educational credits that are limited only by your time and the offerings provided.

Wayne State University offers its Virtual Classroom (Fig. 9.5). This site is a good example of the use of the Internet to deliver basic medical curriculum. With a password and logon ID, buttons allow you to access lecture notes for classes given by various departments. Most of the learning materials are written in HTML and can be viewed directly using an Internet browser, and saved and printed as necessary.

Continuing education is available from consortiums that include smaller universities or those using the term "university" without readily apparent ties to more recognized academic institutions. An example of such a site is the MedConnect CME/CE Center offered by the HealthAtoZ Professional and University of the Sciences in Philadelphia on-line CME/CE center (Fig. 9.6). Use of the site requires registration that is free but does require name, address, e-mail, telephone, date of graduation, and employer information, which not every site requires. Exploration of the site does not readily reveal the exact location, relation, or credentials of the "University of Sciences." This does not mean that the attribution is bogus since a little detective work will lead to the Web site **www.pcps.edu**.

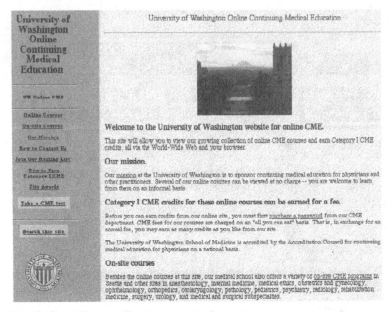

Figure 9.4. The University of Washington offers a mixture of free and fee-based educational opportunities. (**www.uwcme.org**)

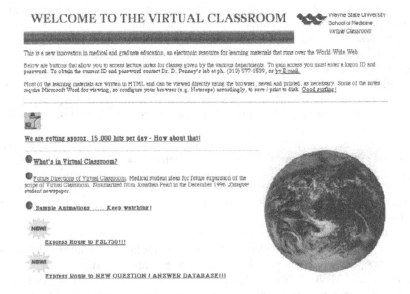

Figure 9.5. The Virtual Classroom is offered by Wayne State University. (**www.phymac.med.wayne.edu/lectpage.htm**)

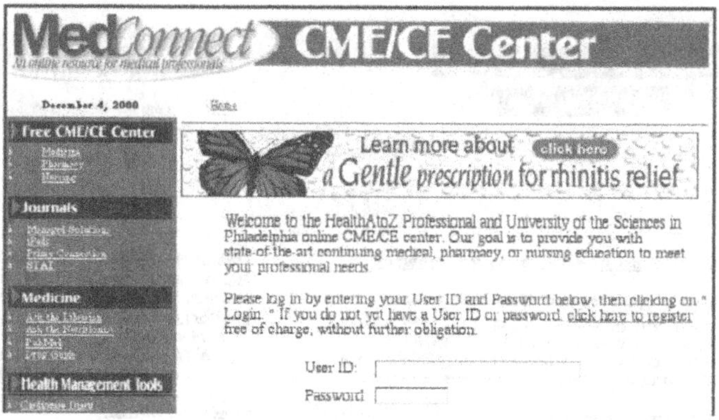

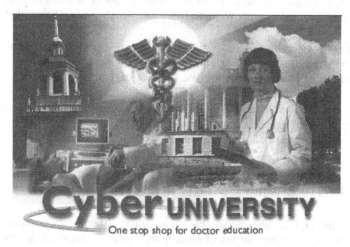

Figure 9.6. The HealthAtoZ Professional and University of the Sciences in Philadelphia on-line CME/CE center offer this continuing education site. (**www.healthatozcme-ce.com/index.html**)

Not all "university" sites are associated with what we normally think of as academic institutions. Cyber University is an example of such a site maintained by a private California corporation (Fig. 9.7). CyberUniversity.net is a portal for medical education for physicians and other health care professionals, offering preparatory exams for undergraduate, graduate, and postgraduate medical education. This includes preparation for specialty board certification and medical licensing. Cyber University offers a range of CME courses that are available on-line, on CD-ROM, video, audio, and text. Cyber University offers courses to prepare for specialty credential exams in 35 medical specialties including anesthesiology, cardiology, neurology, and others.

Continuing education has long been one of the functions of specialty societies in medicine, and on-line continuing education is no exception. Many Inter-

Figure 9.7. The Cyber University offers information on various forms of physician education opportunities. (**www.cyberuniversity.net/PE%20Home.asp**)

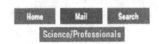

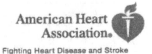

Professional Education

Issues & Controversies In Arrhythmia Management

Products available upon request at no charge: Acute Coronary Syndromes CD-ROM as presented at the 72nd Scientific Sessions and Stroke Education and Slide Lecture Series on CD-ROM. Please email professionaleducation@heart.org to request your complimentary copy of these products.

Coronary Artery Disease in Women: A replay of the 9/16/98 satellite broadcast for physicians and health professionals who treat heart disease.
Note: CME credit NOT available.

ACC/AHA Practice Guidelines

See also Health Professional Education in the Heart and Stroke A-Z Guide.

American Heart Association Monograph Series

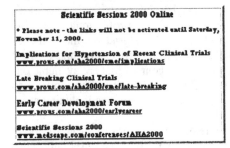

One of the goals of the American Heart Association is to identify and address the educational needs of healthcare professionals in the areas of cardiovascular disease and stroke. The AHA, through the generous support of accredited CME providers, is pleased to offer continuing medical education online.

Additional Online Resources:

Conferences/Meetings

Scientific Sessions

Statements/Guidelines

Research

Councils

Journals

Stroke

Publication

Hypertension Primer, 2nd Edition

Lecture Slide Sets

Figure 9.8. The American Heart Association offers a number of forms of professional continuing education through its Web site. (**www.americanheart.org/ Scientific/CME/**)

net sites maintained by these societies offer their members (and, in some cases, others) opportunities for on-line education. A good example of this type of site is the American Heart Association site (**www.americanheart.org**, Fig. 9.8). In addition to traditional forms of education, the site also offers PowerPoint slide sets that can be downloaded to support other teaching activities. A number of links are provided to other educational materials and opportunities, including information about journals, conferences, and scientific sessions.

Paths to Traditional CME

The Internet, and the sites accessible on it, can be effective in providing pathways to more traditional forms of continuing medical education. Internet sites from national professional organizations, regional societies, and corporate entrepreneurs offer information about upcoming course and educational opportunities. Most offer extended lists of the presenters, topics, and other pertinent information about the offerings. Many of these sites extend the opportunity to register on-line.

At the HELIX Web site, you may order monographs, video programs, and other materials on-line and have them shipped to you. To access the on-line ordering system, you select the "Healthcare Ed Online Catalog" option from the HELIX home page. From that point, you can search for a topic of interest or browse through the catalog. Once you have found items that you'd like to order, you select the "Add to Order" button and follow the instructions to place the order and have items shipped. Most items offered are free of cost (including shipping), though this could change so check your shopping cart carefully.

Medscape, mentioned earlier, offers a continuing medical education calendar with chronologically listed meetings offering traditional educational experiences (Fig. 9.9). The site's database of courses may be searched, but only by geographic region, not by specialty. The site also offers users the ability to compile a list of their CME activities, the date completed, and the credit hours awarded. This can be helpful in complying with state or specialty requirements for education, but the same task can easily be accomplished with a spreadsheet, database, or paper system.

The ability to search efficiently for relevant information is the hallmark of Internet technology. In keeping with this idea, a number of national organizations offer searchable compilations of traditional education opportunities. One of the largest and most authoritative of these sites is the American Medical Association's CME Locator (Fig. 9.10). The over 2,000 AMA-approved educational conferences, seminars, and workshops listed can be searched by specialty, location (U.S., Canada, and international), and dates. These educational programs offer Category 1 activities sponsored by CME providers accredited by the Accreditation Council for Continuing Medical Education (ACCME) or approved

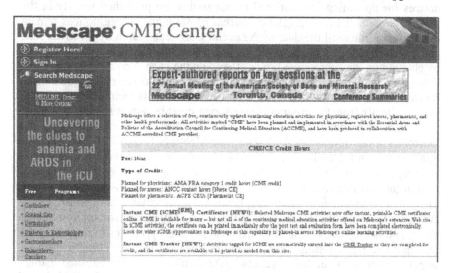

Figure 9.9. Medscape offer a searchable list of continuing medical education offerings. (**www.medscape.com/Home/CMEcenter/CMECenter.html**)

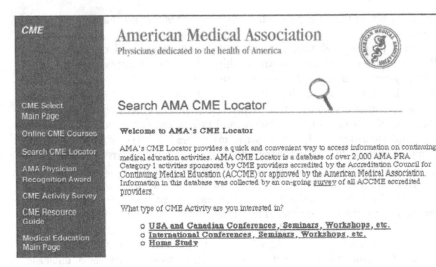

Figure 9.10. The AMA's CME Locator allows users to search for conferences, seminars, and workshops by specialty, location (U.S., Canada, and international), and dates. (**http://www.ama-assn.org/iwcf/iwcfmgr206/cme?**)

by the AMA. These activities provide CME credits that apply toward the AMA Physician Recognition Award and for state or professional society continuing education requirements. Also included at this site are a limited number of approved home study materials that also qualify for CME credits.

The *New England Journal of Medicine* (NEJM) offers a site with links to traditional medical learning opportunities (Fig. 9.11). The NEJM site includes notices for upcoming international meetings that are published weekly in the print version of the *New England Journal of Medicine*. These notices remain available on-line until the date of the event. Users can search by location, date, and keyword to locate meetings of interest. Users can also select the categories by clicking on the appropriate boxes offered on the page. You can click on more than one box in each section or leave the boxes blank to view all of the current notices. The searches at this site are fast, and the results include contact information directly from the program's sponsoring organization or school.

A very large collection of educational opportunities is maintained at the Doctor's Guide to Medical Conference and Meetings (Fig. 9.12). This site lists 5,000 events in the U.S., Canada, and international sites. Like the sites above, meeting information may be searched by subject, date, and location. The site is also organized to make it very easy to view the offerings available in any of more than 36 specialties. These lists, however, are international in scope, so you still have to review the catalog to find those that may be realistic for you to consider. The listings are arranged by date and include hyperlinks to more specific information. These listings are sometimes puzzling in their classification—a search for programs in the "Gynecology/Obstetrics" category returned listings for "International Society for Quality of Life Research Methods Workshops" and "1st Asian International Society for the Study of the Aging Male ISSAM: Meeting on the Aging Male in Kuala Lumpur, Malaysia." Caveat emptor.

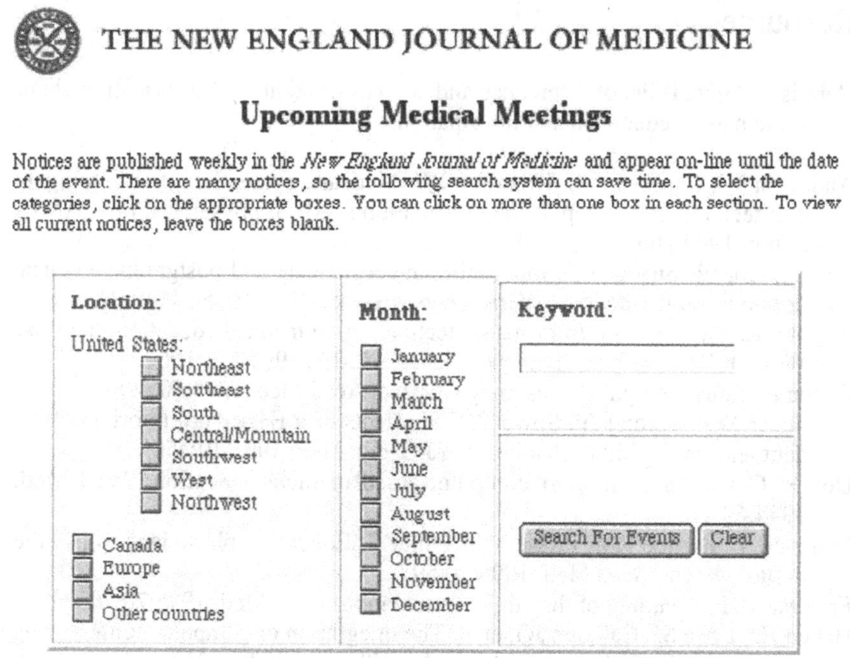
THE NEW ENGLAND JOURNAL OF MEDICINE
Upcoming Medical Meetings
Notices are published weekly in the New England Journal of Medicine and appear on-line until the date of the event. There are many notices, so the following search system can save time. To select the categories, click on the appropriate boxes. You can click on more than one box in each section. To view all current notices, leave the boxes blank.
Location:
United States:
Northeast
Southeast
South
Central/Mountain
Southwest
West
Northwest
Canada
Europe
Asia
Other countries
Month:
January
February
March
April
May
June
July
August
September
October
November
December
Keyword:
Search For Events
Clear

Figure 9.11. The *New England Journal of Medicine* is a traditional location for organizations to publish educational offerings. These are compiled into a collection that can be searched by location, date, and keyword. (**http://www.nejm.org/general/text/Notices.htm**)

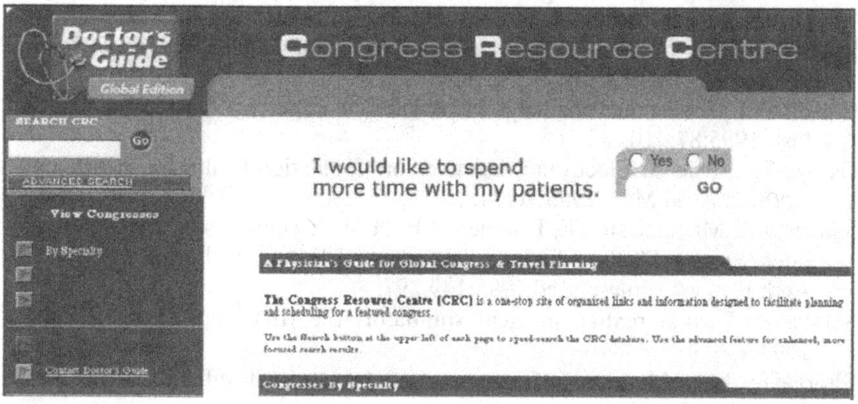
Doctor's Guide
Global Edition
Congress Resource Centre
Go
I would like to spend
more time with my patients.
Yes
No
GO
View Congresses
By Specialty
A Physician's Guide for Global Congress & Travel Planning
Congresses By Specialty

Figure 9.12. The Doctor's Guide to Medical Conference and Meetings site offers information about more than 5,000 possible educational offerings. (**http://www.docguide.com/crc.nsf/web-bySpec**)

Resources

Here is a (limited) list of references and sources of additional information about electronic patient education and information:

Anderson JG, Casebeer LL, Kristofco RE. Medcast: evaluation of an intelligent pull technology to support the information needs of physicians. Proc AMIA Symp. 1999:466.

Bain J, Scott R, Snadden D. Integrating undergraduate and postgraduate education in general practice: experience in Tayside. BMJ. 1995;310:1577.

Bright GR, Hall PW 3rd. Information technology in medical education: the Case Western Reserve University experience. JAMA. 1995;273:1064.

Cohen JJ. Educating physicians in cyberspace. Acad Med. 1995;70:698.

Croninger WR, Tumiel JP, Sowa T. The effects of a Hypercard tutorial on student learning of biomechanics. Am J Occup Ther. 1995;49:456.

Dev P. Consortia to support computer-aided medical education. Acad Med. 1994;69:719.

Florance V, Braude RM, Frisse ME, Fuller S. Educating physicians to use the digital library. Acad Med. 1995;70:597.

Friedman CP. Anatomy of the clinical simulation. Acad Med. 1995;70:205.

Haken JD, Love SJ, Calhoun JG, et al. The integration of computer conferencing into the medical school curriculum. Med Teach. 1989;11:213.

Jaffe CC, Lynch PJ. Computer-aided instruction in radiology: opportunities for more effective learning. Am J Roentgenol. 1995;164:463.

Jerant AF. Training residents in medical informatics. Fam Med. 1999;31:465.

Letterie GS, Morgenstern LL, Johnson L. The role of an electronic mail system in the educational strategies of a residency in obstetrics and gynecology. Obstet Gynecol. 1994;84:137.

Lugo-Vicente H. Internet resources and web pages for pediatric surgeons. Semin Pediatr Surg 2000;9:11.

Nelson C. Libraries face challenge of providing computer access. J Natl Cancer Inst. 1995;87:410.

Ostbye T, Friede A. Electronic resources on population health for a PBL curriculum. Acad Med. 1995;70:748.

Santer DM, Michaelsen VE, Erkonen WE, et al. A comparison of educational interventions. Multimedia textbook, standard lecture, and printed textbook. Arch Pediatr Adolesc Med 1995;149:297.

Satava R. Virtual reality surgical simulator: the first steps. Surg Endosc. 1993;7:203

Shortliffe EH. Medical informatics meets medical education. JAMA. 1995;273:1061, 1064.

Steuer J. Earning CME credit electronically. J Nucl Med. 1999;40(2):9N.

Wofford MM, Wofford JL. The affordability and efficacy of MCAI. Arch Intern Med. 1995;155:1682.

10
Medical Practices and the Web

With all the power that the conjunction of computers and the Internet can provide, why haven't these technologies been rapidly adopted in clinical medicine? Over 80% of physicians use the Internet at home, but this rate drops to one half and one third for office and clinical work areas, respectively[5]. In part, this reluctance has been based on practicality, economics, reliability, speed, and uncertain legal risk. Medical practice is mobile by nature, and until recently there have been few or no alternatives to fixed workstations for medical or Internet applications, limiting point-of-service applications. The economics of medical computing have limited adoption through the associated start-up cost and the lack of an economic benefit from their use. (The main beneficiaries of electronic medical records are institutions or data analysts. Additionally, patient interactions by Internet e-mail is neither reimbursable nor demonstrably more efficient.) Currently available computer and Internet hardware and medical software have a reputation (earned or otherwise) of slow speed and poor reliability. As we will discuss below, even the legal issues of data storage, transmission, and e-mail delivery of health-related information remain unresolved.

Despite these concerns, there are both current and future Internet applications that can enhance the efficiency, efficacy, or ease of some aspects of medical practice. The most obvious areas are those of practice management, practice development and marketing, public and patient relations, and patient interactions (primarily by electronic mail).

---

[5] Harris Interactive national poll of 769 physicians, conducted in the 4th quarter of 1999, reported 3/28/00.

Getting Started (Literally)

The ultimate medical practice application of the Internet is to find a practice in the first place. What was once the province of word-of-mouth, mentor's connections, journal advertising, or the persistence of recruiting firms is becoming a Web-based task. This is not to say that it has replaced the more traditional ways of finding a practice, but it is having a significant impact.

The Internet may be used to search for a medical practice or position in several ways. The Internet is a great tool to obtain general information about a practice or region. Basic demographic data about the medical needs of a community or region can be obtained from sources local to the area, federal agencies, or from specialized information gathered and made available by various specialty societies. Information ranging from housing costs to average rainfall can be on your computer screen in seconds.

Both traditional recruiting firms and new Internet-based physician placement services now populate the Internet. Many professional organizations offer their members job listings or search and placement services. An example of an independent search service is the National TeleAccess Network (NTN) SearchLine (Fig. 10.1). This site is not owned or operated by a commercial search firm or professional recruitment organization. Rather, the site is supported by a consortium of several organizations and financed by advertisers, pharmaceutical companies, and the fees charged to those who list positions available. In operation since 1993, NTN SearchLine provides physicians and health care professionals with a way to carry out their employment searches via the Internet.

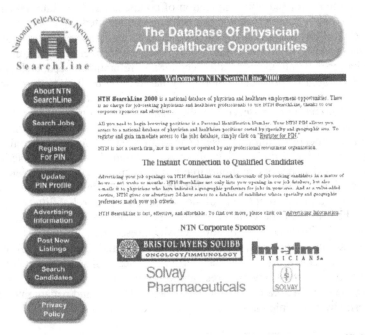

Figure 10.1. The national TeleAccess Network SearchLine allows users to efficiently match up medical employment opportunities and candidates. (**http://ntnjobs.com**)

Practice and Personal Management

The business of medicine is complex and ever changing but vital to the financial survival of the physician and those employed in the industry. The use of computers to facilitate scheduling and billing is hardly new, but a growing number of companies are offering Internet solutions to these tasks. These vary from those who use the Internet simply to access potential buyers and advertise their wares, to those who keep the relevant programs on their systems and provide access (via the Internet) to them as needed (ASP, see glossary). As noted in Chapter 6, many electronic medical record vendors offer systems that are integrated into a complete package for scheduling and billing. If you are considering an electronic record system, such an enhancement is worthwhile. However, the large number of stand-alone scheduling and billing systems available, along with their longer record of experience and reliability, suggests that these systems may serve this function well into the immediate future.

One aspect of medical practice that lends itself well to computer and Internet use is the electronic billing of third-party insurers. This application is especially attractive when combined with an electronic medical record, though this is not automatically included or available in most packages. Based on a recent search of the Internet, software and Internet support for medical billing is available from over 150 vendors or sites (Fig. 10.2). Electronic filing of claims is faster and more direct than paper options. Most software is available for IBM (Windows and DOS) and Macintosh platforms, or (less commonly) directly from an Internet application service provider (ASP).

A number of Internet sites offer medical management tools by way of either Internet connections or as free-standing computer applications. These tools generally allow you to submit reimbursement claims electronically, but also offer additional features designed to enhance productivity or better manage other aspects of your practice. For example, this type of software often allows your staff to check patient insurance eligibility on-line through direct access to payers and their databases of subscribers (Fig. 10.3). Still other sites offer types of support to your office management staff including tailored news articles, e-mail updates, or chat rooms where problems can be shared. Some sites proffer these services in exchange for free registration, while others require fees or licenses. Free sites generally recover the cost of delivering these services through advertising and access to the information you provide about yourself and your practice. (All have privacy policies about the use of patient information, but may not protect your practice information to the same degree.) Internet sites and the information that they supply cannot make up for poor management or organization, but they can be an improvement over paper methods.

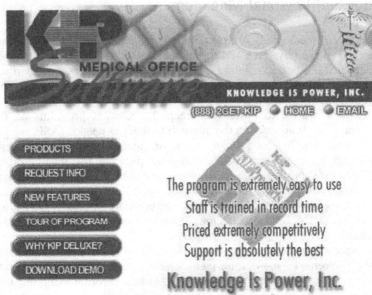

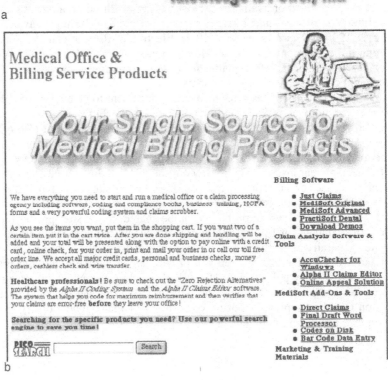

Figure 10.2. Software for electronic medical billing for both the IBM and Macintosh platforms is available from a number of Internet sites. (a, **www.kipdelux.com**; b, **www.new-ventures.com**)

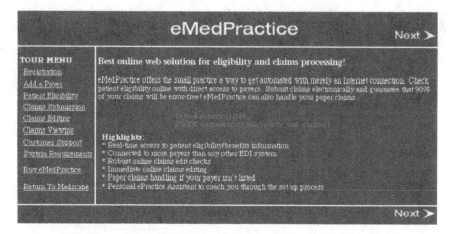

Figure 10.3. Medscape offers eMedPractice medical management software that requires only an Internet connection. (**medoffice.medscape.com/Home/network/MOM/tour/ ePracticeSolutions/slide01.html**)

One new sector of Internet involvement in the arena of management is that of personal information management (PIM). Once the province of paper organizers, or more recently palm-top personal digital assistants (PDAs), a small but growing number of Internet sites offer to perform a similar service. These Internet services will accumulate information that you supply about events, telephone numbers and addresses, to-do lists, and other pieces of information. These replacements for sticky notes, wall calendars, and day planners will display this information in a variety of customizable forms or formats (Fig. 10.4). One of the most useful is a personalized calendar of events sent to your browser when you log on. These sites can also send e-mail or other reminders of important upcoming events (with links to Internet card, flower, or gift vendors) or compare schedules to facilitate meetings between colleagues (if they all use the same service). With your permission, others can enter information or update your schedule. Since the system is Internet based, you can access up-to-date information from any location that offers Internet access. This also means that the information is independent of the platform, allowing various types of computing devices to access the same data.

Beyond just a warehouse of information you provide, these services can also alert you to events or information that may be of interest. For example, you can tell the site about activities you like to do and the agent can inform you of possible activities of interest that are available at the same times you have available. (You could tell a service that you like a particular sport. The server might notice that you have a business trip that places you near a game and provide an alert.) You can book travel on-line and have the travel itinerary added to your daily schedule. Other providers offer sites or PDA programs that act as alarm clocks, reminders, periodic stock updates, or prompts to take medications.

There are a number of suppliers of PIM services. Examples include eDock, Excite Planner, Schedule On-line, SwiftTouch, Visto.com, Yahoo! Calendar,

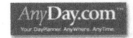

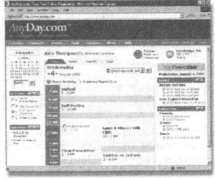

Figure 10.4. Personal Information Managers such as AnyDay.com offer Internet-based tools to manage schedules, events, reminders, and more. (**www.AnyDay.com**)

MyFamily.com, and FamilyBuzz.com. Most pay the cost of their service through advertising revenue raised through their ability to match up seller with potential buyers by virtue of the information you provide. Some providers (AnyDay.com), claim more than 4 million users of their service, providing a substantial market for advertisers.

Practice Development and Promotion

Many practitioners use the Internet to develop and promote their practice. This ranges from a simple Web page to aggressive Internet-based marketing. A recently reported American Medical Association study found that 27% of United States physicians surveyed have their own Web pages.[6] Some practices use electronic mail to send the results of consultation or follow-up to referring physicians or agencies, while others use the Internet to publish informational, educational, or promotional materials for their patients and others. More and more practices feel the need to have a Web page even if they are not sure why.

The most basic form of practice promotion is a simple home page. Examples of Internet Web pages maintained by practices vary from the unadorned to the complex and flashy. Like personal Web pages, most of these are placed on the Internet server of a separate provider (ISP). The information contained is supplied by the practice or physician, but may have been turned into the Web pages

---

[6] *American Medical News*, April 24, 2000, p. 20-1.

by someone in the practice or an outside vendor. The cost of both creating and hosting these Web pages will vary based on the complexity of the page, the size and number of pages, and the pricing structure of the supplier. If you go this route, it pays to shop around. It is also wise to review periodically your involvement with the provider to ensure that you are receiving both the best service and price available.

Some medical associations offer practice Web page development and hosting either directly or through association with other providers. An example of this hybrid is Medem (Fig. 10.5). Medem practice information is linked electronically with the AMA's physician finder system that is also a part of Medem (Fig. 10.6). These listings contain information about the physician, specialty, practice particulars, and even maps and driving directions (Fig. 10.7).

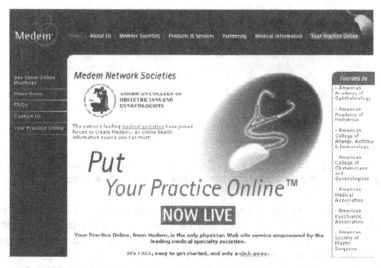

Figure 10.5. Medem offers a both templates and hosting for practice Web pages. (**www.medem.com**)

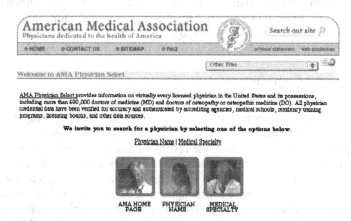

Figure 10.6. The American Medical Association's Physician Finder service uses practice information from Medem when it is available. (**www.ama-assn.org**)

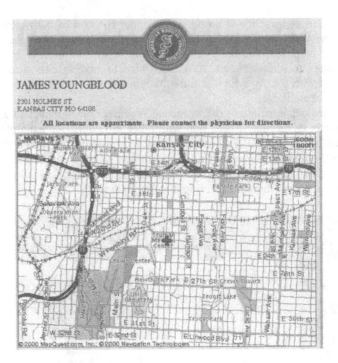

Figure 10.7. When the AMA physician finder is used, driving directions and maps are directly linked and available through a simple click. (**www.ama-assn.org**)

If you use a Web page or pages to promote your practice, it is vital that you periodically review both the page and its content. Changes in Web browser technology or corruption of the electronic file of your page can result in a page that does not load, respond properly, or worse. Having users' computers crash and need to be restarted every time they try to visit your site is not a good reflection on your practice, even though it has nothing to do with the quality of your care. Similarly damning is a page that has outdated information—announcing your holiday closings is a good idea, but only if they are for an upcoming holiday and not one six months ago.

E-mail and Medicine

One aspect of medical practice that would seem to lend itself to computers and the Internet is patient communication. Answering nonacute questions, refilling prescriptions, and communicating the results of laboratory or imaging studies would seem to be logical uses for electronic mail. This would allow you or your staff to address these issues when it is convenient and it can provide a written record for the patient's chart. Your thoughts can be gathered and additional information obtained before replying, resulting in a more complete response. You and your practice have the look and feel of being up to date and well informed. Administrative tasks such as scheduling appointments and treatment reminders are ideally suited for this medium. (Seventy percent of current practice e-mail is for these purposes.) Sounds good. There are, however, some downsides. There are enough concerns that the American Medical Association House of Delegates has adopted guidelines to aid physicians in the appropriate use of e-mail.[7]

One of the greatest concerns about the use of electronic mail for patient communications is privacy. As we have pointed out in earlier chapters, e-mail is neither secure nor private—you have no idea who is reading the message or to whom it will be distributed. Both patients and physicians must be concerned about protecting patient confidentiality, but it is the physician who is legally liable for any breech that may occur. The AMA guidelines suggest that at a minimum, the physician and patient should discuss the use of e-mail and the discussion should be documented in the patient's chart. This could take the form of a written agreement authorizing the use of e-mail between the physician and patient. Most legal advisors also suggest that a privacy statement should be provide on the first page (or a link located on the first page) of any practice's Internet site. Some go so far as to require acceptance of the privacy policy when a patient first registers to use the Web site. Content that should be a part of any privacy statement is outlined in Table 10.1.

Table 10.1 Suggested contents for Web site privacy statement

Identification of information collected
Use of collected information
Distribution of information (if any)
Patient's ability to control collection, use, and distribution of information
A statement of commitment regarding data security
Those steps taken to ensure the quality and security of data
The consequences, if any, of a visitor's refusal to provide information
The accountability of the practice or organization
A method to contact the practice or organization with questions or concerns about privacy

Legislation such as the Health Insurance Portability and Accountability Act of 1996 (HIPAA), and advances in sophisticated authentication systems are establishing guidelines and systems for secure on-line communications between physicians and patients. The new Electronic Signatures in Global and National Commerce Act, known as E-Sign, will make digital signatures as legal as signatures on paper and may help to clear up some privacy issues. These signature systems serve to authenticate the source of the communication, but do not completely resolve the issue of accountability. Also unresolved is the issue of liability and indemnity for such things as lost e-mail, service outages, or technical problems. Until each of these issues is resolved, some general precautions to be followed are shown in Table 10.2.

---

[7] American Medical Association House of Delegates Resolution 810 (A-99), "Guidelines for Patient-Physician Electronic Mail," June 13, 2000.

Table 10.2 E-mail Do's and Don'ts

Do	Don't
Select a form of secure, encrypted e-mail to ensure patient privacy.	Give anonymous advice. Patients (and the physician) must be identified.)
Keep a printed copy of all e-mail (coming and going) in the patient's permanent chart.	Use e-mail for first-time consultations.
Respond promptly to e-mails. (If you said patients could contact you this way, they expect you to follow through.) Messages must be checked and dealt with in timely way.	Refill prescriptions without authenticating the patient's identity.
Address only nonacute issues and conditions.	Delegate the evaluation or response to patient e-mail to anyone else without the patient's permission.
Establish guidelines for acceptable topics (e.g., prescription refills, medical advice, obtaining test results, scheduling appointments, release of records, etc.) and those that are not.	Use e-mail for urgent questions or conditions.
Ask patients to identify the subject or category of their communication in the subject line of the message.	Use group mailings that reveal the name or any other recipient. Even that fact that a patient sees a particular physician or practice is confidential.
Use an automatic reply to indicate that the message has been received and that a response will be sent within a specified period.	Leave open e-mail on an unattended computer.
Let patients know when you have completed a patient-originated request.	Forward e-mail messages with patient-identifiable information without the express permission of the patient.
Give patients an alternative route for follow-up or questions if the e-mail information is insufficient.	Process patient-related e-mail from outside sites.

One partial solution to the issue of privacy in electronic patient communications is being addressed by the secure messaging feature of the Medem Web site. When introduced, secure messaging is a feature that will be available to patients and providers. For physician offices, the feature is available as an option for communication with patients, for communication with their peers, and for patient referral. Once a patient has been approved by the office practice for secure messaging, that patient may initiate a message either from the Medem site or from the provider's custom home page. Patients may select from a set list of subjects for messages, providing boundaries for the type of information dealt with in this way. The secure messaging system provides encryption, authorization, and audit trails that address the security and privacy issues involved. Both the patient and physician's identities are authenticated by the system. The general structure of this system is shown in Fig. 10.8.

An additional issue that has yet to be unraveled is that of medical licensure and the use of electronic mail. Assume your office is located near the border of two states and that you hold a valid medical license in only one. When a patient crosses the state line to come to your office, there are no problems since you (and your practice) are located in the state where you are licensed. As long as the care is furnished in your state (and any prescriptions provided are filled there as well), there are no issues. What is unclear is the legality of providing medical advice or treatment when these are rendered in the patient's home using the Internet. Does this constitute practicing in that state? You could argue that this is just an extension of your office and no different than if the patient had placed a telephone call to your office. The question is murkier if the states are not contiguous or if you do not already have a doctor-patient relationship established. Most states consider the place of residence of the patient to be the determining factor in determining where the practice of medicine took place. Many states allow an unlicensed physician to consult with another physician (but not the patient), including teleradiology and teleconferencing. Some states,[8] however, do not consider e-mail or telephone conversations to be telemedicine, and are therefore exempt. Until some national consensus and coordination of existing laws occur, no clear guidelines are possible.

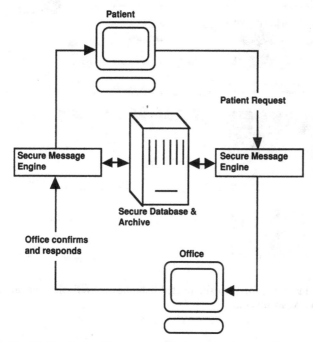

Figure 10.8. The Medex Secure Messaging system uses an intermediate message engine and data archive to authenticate and encrypt doctor-patient communications.

---

[8] At the time of this writing, California is one such state.

Pitfalls and Provisos

As noted above, there are a number of concerns specific to the Internet and medical practice. These range from the licensure issues related to telemedicine and medical e-mail, to special liabilities related to materials published on your practice's Internet site. Yes, you can be held liable for statements made on your Web site in the same way that you would be for other published statements. Breeches in security, loss of information, and other uncharted legal hazards are waiting to place you at risk. There has even grown up a thriving industry for Internet and Web page insurance (Fig. 10.9). The risks associated with Web pages and an Internet medical presence are both real and still being defined. If you are going to use the power of the Internet for medical practice tasks, you would be wise to consult legal counsel and watch authoritative sources for information about this evolving area.

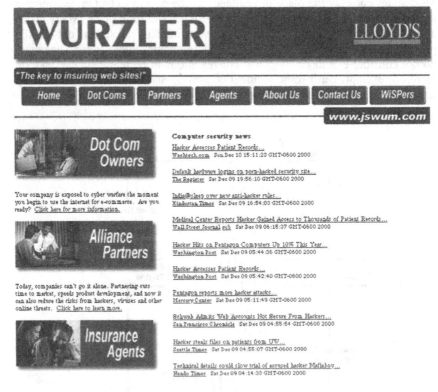

Figure 10.9. Insurance for Web site-related liabilities is available from any number of providers. (**www.jswum.com**)

Resources

Here is a (limited) list of references and sources of additional information about electronic patient education and information:

Borowitz SM, Wyatt JC. The origin, content, and workload of e-mail consultations. JAMA. 1998;280:1321.

Christmas WA, Turner HS, Crothers L. Should college health providers use e-mail to communicate with their patients? Two points of view. J Am Coll Health. 2000;49:39-43.

Ellis JE, Klock PA, Mingay DJ, Roizen MF. Use of electronic mail for postoperative follow-up after ambulatory surgery. J Clin Anesth. 1999;11:136-9.

Eysenbach G, Diepgen TL. Responses to unsolicited patient e-mail requests for medical advice on the World Wide Web. JAMA. 1998;280:1333.

Kane B, Sands DZ. Guidelines for the clinical use of electronic mail with patients. The AMA Internet Working Group, Task Force on Guidelines for the Use of Clinic-Patient Electronic Mail. J Am Med Inform Assoc. 1998;5:104-11.

Spielberg AR. On call and on-line. JAMA. 1998;280:1353-9.

Vogelsmeier SJ. E-mail communications with patients. Missouri Med. 2000;97:507-8.

Appendix 1
Sources of Additional Information

Adams PC, Gregor JC, Kertesz AE, Valberg LS. Screening blood donors for hereditary hemochromatosis: decision analysis model based on a 30-year database. Gastroenterology. 109:177, 1995

Agho AO, Williams AM. Actual and desired computer literacy among allied health students. J Allied Health. 24:117, 1995

Allen J. Surgical Internet at a glance: hand surgery and transplantation. Am J Surg. 179:431, 2000

Anderson RK, Haddix A, McCray JC, Wunz TP. Developing a health information infrastructure for Arizona. Bull Med Libr Assoc. 82:396, 1994

Anonymous. Maximum Security. A Hacker's Guide to Protecting Your Internet Site and Network. Indianapolis: Sams Publishing, 1997.

Anthes DL, Berry RE, Lanning A. Internet resources for family physicians. Canadian Family Physician. 43:1104, 1997

Bailes JE. Present technology and future applications. Clin Neurosurg. 45:192-201, 1999

Bain J, Scott R, Snadden D. Integrating undergraduate and postgraduate education in general practice: experience in Tayside. Br Med J. 310:1577, 1995

Barnett GO, Justice NS. COSTAR—a computer-based medical information system for medical care. Proc IEEE. 67:1226, 1979

Barnett GO. The computer and clinical judgement. N Engl J Med. 307:493, 1982

Barry MJ, Fowler FJ Jr, Mulley AG Jr, Henderson JV Jr, Wennberg JE. Patient reactions to a program designed to facilitate patient participation in treatment decisions for benign prostatic hyperplasia. Med Care (Phila). 33:771, 1995

Baumlin KM, Bessette MJ, Lewis C, Richardson LD. EM. CyberSchool. an evaluation of computer-assisted instruction on the Internet. Acad Emerg Med. 7:959-62, 2000

Belinson JL, McClure MS, Deutsch RA. A new automated tumor registry and clinical research system and its application to gynecology oncology patients. Gynecol Oncol. 27:264, 1987

Bell DS, Fonarow GC, Hays RD, Mangione CM. Self-study from Web-based and printed guideline materials. A randomized, controlled trial among resident physicians. Ann Intern Med. 132:938-46, 2000

Bell T. Internet for the allergist. J Asthma. 33:143, 1996

Benedicto PJ. The information age: what's it all about? J Med Assoc Ga. 84:117, 1995

Benger J. A review of telemedicine in accident and emergency: the story so far. J Accid Emerg Med. 17:157-64, 2000

Bergman R. Where there's a will—computer-based patient records require commitment, time—and money. Hosp Health Netw. 68:36, 1994

Berner ES, Webster GD, Shugerman AA, et al. Performance of four computer-based diagnostic systems. N Engl J Med. 330:1792, 1994

Bigby JA, Giblin J, Pappius E, et al. Appointment reminders to reduce no-show rates: a stratified analysis of their cost-effectiveness. JAMA. 250:1742, 1983

Binik YM, Servan-Schreiber D. Intelligent computer-based assessment and psychotherapy. An expert system for sexual dysfunction. J Nerv Ment Dis. 176:387, 1988

Bishara SE, Cummins DM, Jorgensen GJ, Jakobsen JR. A computer-assisted photogrammetric analysis of soft tissue changes after orthodontic treatment. Part I: methodology and reliability. Am J Orthod Dentofacial Orthop. 107:633, 1995

Borowitz SM, Wyatt JC. The origin, content, and workload of e-mail consultations. JAMA. 280:1321, 1998

Brahmi FA. MEDLINE, CANCER-CD, SCI-CD addition on CD-ROM. MD Comput. 6:12, 1989

Braude RM, Florance V, Frisse M, Fuller S. The organization of the digital library. Acad Med. 70:286, 1995

Briggs JS. Measuring the readership of a health-related Website. J Telemed Telecare. 6 (suppl 2):S2-5, 2000

Bright GR, Hall PW III. Information technology in medical education: the Case Western Reserve University experience. JAMA. 273:1064, 1995

Briley MS, Hoare M, Dobson D, Anslow PL. Imlink and continuing medical education: the use of an image transfer system to broadcast teaching cases nationally. Br J Radiol. 67:453, 1994

Brown LJ, Caldwell SB, Eklund SA. How fee and insurance changes could affect dentistry: results from a microsimulation model. J Am Dent Assoc. 126:449, 1995

Butow PN, Dunn SM, Tattersall MH, Jones QJ. Computer-based interaction analysis of the cancer consultation. Br J Cancer. 71:1115, 1995

Capusten B. Continuing professional development for radiologists using the Web as a delivery vehicle. J Digit Imaging. 13(2 suppl 1):54-5, 2000

Catanzarite VA, Jelovsek FR. What's the best role for computer-aided instruction? Contemp Obstet Gynecol. 34:65, 1989

Chadwick DW, Crook PJ, Young AJ, McDowell DM, Dornan TL, New JP. Using the Internet to access confidential patient records: a case study. BMJ. 321:612-4, 2000

Channin DS. Radiology and the Internet. Acad Radiol. 2:721, 1995

Chard T. Human versus machine: a comparison of a computer "expert system" with human experts in the diagnosis of vaginal discharge. Int J Biomed Comput. 20:71, 1987

Cheswick W, Bellovin SM. How computer security works: firewalls. Sci Am. 279(4):106, 1998

Chilton L, Berger JE, Melinkovich P, et al. American Academy of Pediatrics. Pediatric Practice Action Group and Task Force on Medical Informatics.

Privacy protection and health information: patient rights and pediatrician responsibilities. Pediatrics. 104:973-7, 1999

Chi-Lum BI, Lundberg GD, Silberg WM. Physicians accessing the Internet, the PAI Project: an educational initiative. JAMA. 275:1361, 1996

Christmas WA, Turner HS, Crothers L. Should college health providers use e-mail to communicate with their patients? Two points of view. J Am Coll Health. 49:39-43, 2000

Cimino JJ. Beyond the superhighway: exploiting the Internet with medical informatics. J Am Med Informatics Assoc. 4:279, 1997

Clark R, Geller B, Peluso N, McVety D, Worden JK. Development of a community mammography registry: experience in the breast screening program project. Radiology. 196:811, 1995

Cohen JJ. Educating physicians in cyberspace. Acad Med. 70:698, 1995

Cohn MJ, Cohen AJ. RADCOM: a computerized translation device for use during fluoroscopic examination of non-English-speaking patients. Am J Roentgenol. 162:455, 1994

Corn M, Johnson FE. Connecting the health sciences community to the Internet: the NLM/NSF grant program. Bull Med Libr Assoc. 82:392, 1994

Cosyns B. Internet in cardiology: a new toy or a new tool? Acta Cardiol. 54:253-5, 1999

Cristoforoni PM, Gerbaldo D, Perino A, Piccoli R, Montz FJ, Capitanio GL. Computerized colposcopy: results of a pilot study and analysis of its clinical relevance. Obstet Gynecol. 85:1011, 1995

Croninger WR, Tumiel JP, Sowa T. The effects of a Hypercard tutorial on student learning of biomechanics. Am J Occup Ther. 49:456, 1995

Daly J, Fletcher J, Herbig F, et al The use of the Laser video disc/computer system in medical education. In Blum BI (ed): Proceedings of the 6th Annual Symposium on Computer Applications in Medical Care, p 1011. Silver Spring, MD: IEEE Computer Society Press, 1982

Dawson R, Gilbertson J, Kim S, Becich M. Pathology imaging on the Web. Extending the role of the pathologist as educator to patients. Clin Lab Med. 19:849-66, 1999

DeCherney GS. Web-based medicine. Del Med J. 72:289-91, 2000

Della Mea V. Internet electronic mail: a tool for low-cost telemedicine. J Telemed Telecare. 5:84-9, 1999

Dev P. Consortia to support computer-aided medical education. Acad Med. 69:719, 1994

Diaz J, Miranda OM, Faundes A, et al. Preliminary experiment with computerized anamnesis in gynecology and reproductive health. Int J Gynaecol Obstet. 24:285, 1986

Dieu T, Donahoe SR. Digital camera and the Internet: bringing the patient home. Med J Aust. 171:567, 1999

Dini EF, Linkins RW, Chaney M. Effectiveness of computer-generated telephone messages in increasing clinic visits. Arch Pediatr Adolesc Med. 149:902, 1995

Doupi P, van der Lei J. Rx medication information for the public and the WWW: quality issues. Med Inform Internet Med. 24:171-9, 1999

Downie AC. Teaching radiology on the Internet. Clin Radiol. 52:4, 1997

Doyle DJ. New media. Can J Anaesth. 47:474-6, 2000

Duisterholt JS, Schoemaker J. AIDA for reproductive medicine and the fertility clinic. Comput Methods Programs Biomed. 25:305, 1987

Dutcher GA, Arnesen SJ. Developing a subject-specific Gopher at the National Library of Medicine. Bull Med Libr Assoc. 83:228, 1995

Eddings J. How the Internet Works. Emeryville, CA: Ziff-Davis Press, 1994

Elkind A, Eardley A, Haran D, Spencer B, Smith A. Computer-managed call and recall for cervical screening: a typology of reason for non-attendance. Community Med. 11:157, 1989

El-Shazly M, Maiwald G. The Internet: a new friend to plastic surgeons. Plast Reconstr Surg. 106:235-6, 2000

Engelmeir KH, Poppl SJ. A new imaging method and its application in gynecological treatment planning. In Salamon R, Blum BI, Jorgensen M (eds). Proceedings of the 5th Conference of Medical Informatics, p 475. Amsterdam: Elsevier, 1986

Evans RS, Pestotnik SL, Classen DC, Horn SD, Bass SB, Burke JP. Preventing adverse drug events in hospitalized patients. Ann Pharmacother. 28:523, 1994

Evers WM. Are patient smart cards the right way to go? No. Hosp Health Netw. 68:10, 1994

Eysenbach G, Diepgen TL. Responses to unsolicited patient e-mail requests for medical advice on the World Wide Web. JAMA. 280:1333, 1998

Feingold M, Kewalramani R, Kaufmann GE. Internet and obstetrics and gynecology. Acta Obstet Gynecol Scand. 76:718, 1997

Feldman MD. Munchausen by Internet: detecting factitious illness and crisis on the Internet. South Med J. 93:669-72, 2000

Ferguson T. Digital doctoring—opportunities and challenges in electronic patient-physician communication. JAMA. 280:1361, 1998

Fikar CR. The Internet and the pediatrician: should there be a connection? Clin Pediatr. 35:229, 1996

Fine J, Ashwood ER, Adams JS. Computer-video laser disc systems: applications in medicine. In Lindberg DA, Collen MF, Van Brunt EE (eds): Proceedings AMIA Congress, 1982, p 188. New York: Masson, 1982

Flahault A, Dias-Ferrao V, Chaberty P, Esteves K, Valleron A-J, Lavanchy D. FluNet as a tool for global monitoring of influenza on the Web. JAMA. 280:1330, 1998

Flets WD. Classification standards for billing databases and health-care reimbursement. MD Comput. 5:20, 1988

Florance V, Braude RM, Frisse ME, Fuller S. Educating physicians to use the digital library. Acad Med. 70:597, 1995

Ford W. How computer security works: digital certificates. Sci Am. 279(4):108, 1998

Frank MS, Johnson JA. Computerized tracking of mammography patients: value of a radiology information system integrated with a personal-computer data base. Am J Roentgenol. 163:705, 1994

Frasca D, Malezieux R, Mertens P, Neidhardt JP, Voiglio EJ. Review and evaluation of anatomy sites on the Internet. Surg Radiol Anat. 22:107-10, 2000

Friedman CP. Anatomy of the clinical simulation. Acad Med. 70:205, 1995

Frisse ME, Schnase JL, Metcalfe ES. Models for patient records. Acad Med. 69:546, 1994

Fuller SS. Internet connectivity for hospitals and hospital libraries: strategies. Bull Med Libr Assoc. 83:32, 1995

Furness PN. The use of digital images in pathology. J Pathol. 183:253, 1997

Gibbons PS, Pishotta FT, Stepto RC. A system for reporting gynecologic procedures: a linguistic-logic approach. J Reprod Med. 28:201, 1983

Glowniak J. The Internet as an information source for geriatricians. Drugs & Aging. 10:169, 1997

Gobis LJ. Computerized patient records. Start preparing now. J Nurs Admin. 24:15, 1994

Golder DT, Brennan KA. Practicing dentistry in the age of telemedicine. J Am Dent Assoc. 131:734-44, 2000

Gomella LG. The Wild, Wild Web: resources for counseling patients with prostate cancer in the Information Age. Semin Urol Oncol. 18:167-71, 2000

Gosling J. How computer security works: the Java sandbox. Sci Am. 279(4):109, 1998

Greaves DR. Immunology on the Internet. Curr Opinion Immunol. 9:449, 1997

Gross GW, Boone JM, Bishop DM. Pediatric skeletal age: determination with neural networks. Radiology. 195:689, 1995

Grunfeld A, Ho K. An Internet primer, part II: tools of the Internet. J Emerg Med. 15:401, 1997

Guillerman RP. Evaluating online radiology information resources. Acad Radiol. 6:561-2, 1999

Hahn H, Stout R. The Internet Complete Reference. Berkeley, CA: Osborne McGraw-Hill, 1994

Hahn H, Stout R. The Internet Yellow Pages, 2nd ed. Berkeley, CA: Osborne McGraw-Hill, 1995

Hahn PF, Lee MJ, Gazelle GS, Forman BH, Mueller PR. A simplified Hyper-Card data base for patient management in an interventional practice: experience with more than 4000 cases. Am J Roentgenol. 162:1443, 1994

Ham HR, Rozenberg S. Information on nuclear medicine tests on the Internet. Nucl Med Commun. 21:308, 2000

Hammond WE, Stead WW, Straube MJ, et al. Functional characteristics of a computerized medical record. Methods Inf Med. 19:157, 1980

Hasley S. A comparison of computer-based and personal interviews for the gynecologic history update. Obstet Gynecol. 85:494, 1995

Hawkins RS. Medical information systems and their importance in managed care. Gastroenterol Clin North Am. 26:823, 1997

Herxheimer A, McPherson A, Miller R, Shepperd S, Yaphe J, Ziebland S. Database of patients' experiences (DIPEx): a multi-media approach to sharing experiences and information. Lancet. 355(9214):1540-3, 2000

Hody GL, Avner RA. The PLATO system: An evaluative description. In DeLand ED (ed): Information Technology in Health Science Education, p 143. New York: Plenum, 1978

Hollander SM, Lanier D. Orientation to the Internet for primary care health professionals. Bull Med Libr Assoc. 83:96, 1995

Hopper KD, Zajdel M, Hulse SF, et al. Interactive method of informing patients of the risks of intravenous contrast media. Radiology. 192:67, 1994

Horowitz GL, Jackson JD, Bleich HL. PaperChase: self-service bibliographic retrieval. JAMA. 250:2494, 1983

Horsch A, Balbach T, Melnitzki S, Knauth J. Learning tumor diagnostics and medical image processing via the WWW—the case-based radiological textbook ODITEB. Int J Med Inf. 58-59:39-50, 2000

Hubbs PR, Rindfleisch TC, Godin P, Melmon KL. Medical information on the Internet. JAMA. 280:1363, 1998

Huntley AC. Dermatology Online Journal: an Internet-based journal for dermatologists. Int J Dermatol. 36:577, 1997

Institute of Medicine, Committee on Improving the Patient Record. The Computer-Based Patient Record: An Essential Technology for Health Care. Washington, DC: National Academy Press, 1991

Jadad AR, Gagliardi A. Rating health information on the Internet: navigating to knowledge or to Babel? JAMA. 279:611, 1998

Jadad AR, Haynes RB, Hunt D, Browman GP. The Internet and evidence-based decision-making: a needed synergy for efficient knowledge management in health care. CMAJ. 162:362-5, 2000

Jaffe CC, Lynch PJ. Computer-aided instruction in radiology: opportunities for more effective learning. Am J Roentgenol. 164:463, 1995

Jelovsek FR. Application of computer technology to reproductive endocrinology. Clin Obstet Gynecol. 32:605, 1989

Jelovsek FR. Microcomputer-aided instruction for ob/gyn education. J Perinat Med. 16:339, 1988

Jelovsek FR, Deason BP, Richard H. Impact of an on-line information system on patients and personnel in the medical office. In Blum BI (ed): Proceedings of the 6th Annual Symposium on Computer Applications in Medical Care, p 85. Silver Spring, MD: IEEE Computer Society Press, 1982

Jelovsek FR, Hammond WE, Stad WW, et al. Computer base reports for ambulatory care administration management. In Lindberg DA, Collen MF, Van Brunt EE (eds): Proceedings of the AMIA Congress, 1982, p 10. New York: Masson, 1982

Jelovsek FR, Rittwage J, Pearse WH, et al. Information management needs of the obstetrician/gynecologist: a survey. Obstet Gynecol. 73:395, 1989

Jerome LW, DeLeon PH, James LC, Folen R, Earles J, Gedney JJ. The coming of age of telecommunications in psychological research and practice. Am Psychol. 55:407-21, 2000

Kahan SE, Seftel AD, Resnick MI. Sildenafil and the Internet. J Urol. 163:919-23, 2000

Kalra D. Electronic health records: the European scene. Br Med. J 309:1358, 1994

Kassirer J. A report card on computer-assisted diagnosis—the grade: C. N Engl J Med. 330:1824, 1994

Kassirer JD, Angell M. The Internet and the journal. N Engl J Med. 332:1709, 1995

Keith RDF, Beckley S, Garibaldi JM, Westgate JA, Ifeachor EL, Greene KR. A multicenter comparative study of 17 experts and an intelligent computer system for managing labor using the cardiotocogram. Br J Obstet Gynaecol. 102:688, 1995

Kienzle M, Curry D, Franken EA Jr, et al. Iowa's National Laboratory for the study of rural telemedicine: a description of a work in progress. Bull Med Libr Assoc. 83:37, 1995

Killeen AA. Overview of current Internet resources for molecular pathology. J Clin Lab Anal 10:375, 1996

Kingsnorth A. eSurgery. Ann R Coll Surg Engl. 82(6 suppl):191-3, 2000

Klein MS, Ross FV, Adams DL, Gilbert CM. Effect of online literature searching on length of stay and patient care costs. Acad Med. 69:489, 1994

Kramer JM, Cath A. Medical resources and the internet. Making the connection. Arch Intern Med. 156:833, 1996

Krejci-Papa NC, Bittorf A, Diepgen T, Huntley A. Dermatology on the Internet. A source of clinical and scientific information. J Dermatol Sci. 13:1, 1996

Kronz JD, Silberman MA, Allsbrook WC, Epstein JI. A Web-based tutorial improves practicing pathologists' gleason grading of images of prostate carcinoma specimens obtained by needle biopsy. Cancer. 89:1818-23, 2000

Krysztoforski J. Are patient smart cards the right way to go? Yes. Hosp Health Netw. 68:10, 1994

Kunkel EJ, Myers RE, Lartey PL, Oyesanmi O. Communicating effectively with the patient and family about treatment options for prostate cancer. Urol Oncol. 18:233-40, 2000

Lacher D, Nelson E, Bylsma W, Spena R. Computer use and needs of internists: a survey of members of the American College of Physcians—American Society of Internal Medicine. Proc AMIA Symp. (20 suppl):453-6, 2000

Lacroix EM, Backus JE, Lyon BJ. Service providers and users discover the Internet. Bull Med Libr Assoc. 82:412, 1994

Lau RK. Genitourinary medicine and the Internet, no. 4. Genitourinary Med. 73:73, 1997

Lau RK. Genitourinary medicine and the Internet, no 5. Genitourinary Med. 73:144, 1997

Leong SL, Baldwin CD, Usatine RP, Adelman AM, Gjerde CL. Web-based education in family medicine predoctoral programs. Fam Med. 32:696-700, 2000

Lepper PC, Margulis EB. Multi-user physician workstation for obstetrics and gynecology: a prototype. In Blum BI (ed): Proceedings of the 9th Annual Symposium on Computer Applications in Medical Care, p 492. Silver Spring, MD: IEEE Computer Society Press, 1985

Letterie GS, Morgenstern LL, Johnson L. The role of an electronic mail system in the educational strategies of a residency in obstetrics and gynecology. Obstet Gynecol 84:137, 1994

Leung KS, Wong FW, Lam W. The development of an expert computer system on medical consultation. Int J Biomed Comput 23:265, 1988

Levine JR, Baroudi C. The Internet for Dummies. San Mateo, CA: IDG Books Worldwide, 1993

Levine JR, Young ML. More Internet for Dummies. San Mateo, CA: IDG Books Worldwide, 1994

Lilford RJ, Glyn-Evans D, Chard T. The use of a patient interactive microcomputer system to obtain histories in an infertility and gynecologic endocrinology clinic. Am J Obstet Gynecol. 146:374, 1983

Lim PH. The urologist and the Internet. Br J Urol. 80 (suppl 3):2, 1997

Lindberg DA. HPCC and the National Information Infrastructure: an overview. Bull Med Libr Assoc. 83:29, 1995

Lindberg DA, Humphreys BL. Computers in medicine. JAMA. 273:1667, 1995

Lindberg DAB. Use of MEDLINE by physicians for clinical problem solving. JAMA. 269:3124, 1993

Lindberg DAB, Humphreys BL. Medicine and health on the Internet: the good, the bad, and the ugly. JAMA. 280:1303, 1998

Lindberg DAB, Siegel ER, Rapp BA, Wallingford KT, Wilson SR. Use of MEDLINE by physicians for clinical problem solving. JAMA. 269:3124, 1993

Liu D. WebCat: the library catalogue on the world wide web. Ann R Coll Surg Engl. 81(7 suppl):324-5, 1999

Lowe HJ, Lomax EC, Polonkey SE. The World Wide Web: a review of an emerging Internet-based technology for the distribution of biomedical information. J Am Med Informatics Assoc. 3:1, 1996

Ludwig M. The Giant Black Book of Computer Viruses, 2nd ed. Show Low, AZ: American Eagle Publications, 1998

Lundberg GD, for the JAMA Review Group. One multimedial medical world. JAMA. 274:655, 1995

Maddison I. The Internet and radiology. Br J Radiol. 70 Spec No:S194, 1997

Mak V. Radiology on the Internet. Hosp Med. 61:291, 2000

Malakoff G, Pincetl PS, el-Bayoumi J, Chang L, Piemme TE. Computer-based patient simulations and their effect on standardized-test scores during a medicine clerkship. Acad Med. 69:155, 1994

Marra CA, Carleton BC, Lynd LD, et al. Drug and poison information resources on the Internet, Part 2: identification and evaluation. Pharmacotherapy 16:806, 1996

Matheson NW. The idea of the library in the twenty-first century. Bull Med Libr Assoc 83:1, 1995

Mawer GE, Lucas SB, Knowles BR, et al. Computer-assisted prescribing of kanamycin for patients with renal insufficiency. Lancet. 1:23, 1972

Mayo WA. Computing & technology. Optometry. 71:196-7, 2000

McDonald CJ. Protocol-based computer reminders, the quality of care and the non-perfectibility of man. N Engl J Med. 295:1351, 1976

McDonald CJ, Overhage JM, Dexter PR, et al. Canopy computing: using the Web in clinical practice. JAMA. 280:1325, 1998

McEnery KW. The Internet, World-Wide Web, and Mosaic: an overview. Am J Roentgenol. 164:469, 1995

McEwen JE. Forensic DNA data banking by state crime laboratories. Am J Hum Genet. 56:1487, 1995

Meinel CP. How hackers break in... and how they are caught. Sci Am. 279(4):98, 1998

Miller RA, Pople HE Jr, Myers JD. INTERNIST-I, an experimental computer-based diagnostic consultant for general internal medicine. N Engl J Med. 307:468, 1982

Millman A, Lee N, Kealy K. ABC of medical computing. The Internet BMJ. 311:440, 1995

Mitchell P. E-prescribing. All dosed up. Health Serv J. Mar. 16;110(5696):suppl 6-7, 2000

Montague J. Serious fun. Zap! Zowie! Pow! Hosp Health Netw. 69:52, 1995

Montbriand MJ. Decision tree model describing alternate health care choices made by oncology patients. Cancer Nurs. 18:104, 1995

Mooney GA, Bligh JG. Information technology in medical education: current and future applications. Postgrad Med. J 73:701, 1997

Nadler GL. Computerized imaging, is it for you? Am J Orthod Dentofacial Orthop. 107:106, 1995

Nelson C. Libraries face challenge of providing computer access. J Natl Cancer Inst. 87:410, 1995

Neurath PW, Enslein K, Mitchell GW. Design of a computer system to assist in differential diagnosis for pelvic surgery. N Engl J Med. 280: 745, 1969

Norman J. Building the computer-based patient record. JAMA. 273:1063, 1995

O'Reilly M. The future is now as the electronic transfer of patient files, images and lab results begins. Can Med Assoc J. 151:1312, 1994

Ornstein S, Bearden A. Patient perspectives on computer-based medical records. J Fam Pract. 38:606, 1994

Osburn AE, Neches NM, Shissler GE, et al. Enhancement of COSTAR with a problem- oriented record structure and decision making support functions. In Hefferman SJ (ed): Proceedings of the 5th Annual Symposium on Computer Applications in Medical Care, p 1011. Silver Spring, MD: IEEE Computer Society Press, 1982

Osman LM, Abdalla MI, Beattie JA, et al. Reducing hospital admission through computer supported education for asthma patients. Grampian Asthma Study of Integrated Care (GRASSIC). Br Med J. 308:568, 1994

Ostbye T, Friede A. Electronic resources on population health for a PBL curriculum. Acad Med. 70:748, 1995

Ouellette F. Internet resources for the clinical geneticist. Clin Genet. 56:179-85, 1999

Overhage JM, Tierney WM, McDonald CJ. Design and implementation of the Indianapolis Network for Patient Care and Research. Bull Med Libr Assoc. 83:48, 1995

Pallen M. Electronic mail. BMJ. 311:1487, 1995

Pallen M. Guide to the Internet. The World Wide Web. BMJ. 311:1552, 1995

Pallen M. Introducing the Internet. BMJ. 311:1422, 1995

Pallen MJ. Medicine and the Internet: dreams, nightmares and reality. Br J Hosp Med. 56:506, 1996

Paperny DM. Computers and information technology: implications for the 21st century. Adolesc Med. 11:183-202, 2000

Perednia DA, Brown NA. Teledermatology: one application of telemedicine. Bull Med Libr Assoc. 83:42, 1995

Perez JC, McKeller MR, Perez JC, Sanchez EE, Ramirez MS. An Internet database of crotaline venom found in the United States. Toxicon. May 1;39:621-632, 2001

Peters R, Sikorski R. Building your own: a physician's guide to creating a Web site. JAMA. 280, 1365, 1998

Pike MA. Special Edition Using the Internet, 2nd ed. Indianapolis, IN: Que Corporation, 1995

Powsner SM, Tufte ER. Graphical summary of patient status. Lancet. 344:386, 1994

Prasad S. Internet mailing lists: a primer. J R Coll Surg Edinb. 45:122-6, 2000

Raines JR, Ellis LBM. A conversational microcomputer-based health risk appraisal. Comput Methods Programs Biomed. 14:175, 1982

Rauch S, Holt MC, Horner M, Rambo N. Community hospitals and the Internet: lessons from pilot connections. Bull Med Libr Assoc. 82:401, 1994

Rawn C, Davidon R, Meier A. Using Web-based case presentations to supplement a surgery clerkship curriculum. Acad Med. 75:540, 2000

Regennitter FJ, Volz JE. An introduction to the Internet. Am J Orthod Dentofacial Orthop. 107:214, 1995

Reino AJ, Rothschild M, Lawson W. Enhanced photodocumentation using photo CD imaging and computer color output. Laryngoscope. 105:556, 1995

Riss P, Radivojevic K. Classification and documentation of vulvar changes: organization of a data bank by personal computer. Geburtsh Frauenheilkd. 49:728, 1989

Riss PA, Koelbl H, Reinthaller A, Deutinger J. Development and application of simple expert systems in obstetrics and gynecology. J Perinat Med. 16:283, 1988

Rivest RL. The case against regulating encryption technology. Sci Am. 279(4):116, 1998

Robertson AJ, Reid GS, Stoker CA, et al. Evaluation of a call programme for cervical cytology screening in women aged 50–60. Br Med J Clin Res. 299:163, 1989

Robinson TN, Partick K, Eng TR, Gustafson D, for the Science Panel on Interactive Communications and Health: An evidence-based approach to interactive health communication. JAMA. 280:1264, 1998

Rock JA, Early SA, Zacur HA, et al. A computer-based system for patient care and research management in reproductive endocrinology. Fertil Steril. 45:216, 1986

Ryan D, Waterston R. Transforming continuing education materials for on-line learning. J Telemed Telecare. 6 (suppl 2):S64-6, 2000

Safran C, Rind DM, Davis RB, et al. Guidelines for management of HIV infection with computer-based patient's record. Lancet. 346:341, 1995

Sandler MP. PubMed central: the JNM perspective. J Nucl Med. 41:1123-4, 2000

Sandroni S, McGee J. The digital toolbox for teaching. South Med J. 88:1199, 1995

Santer DM, D'Alessandro MP, Huntley JS, Erkonen WE, Galvin JR. The multimedia textbook. A revolutionary tool for pediatric education. Arch Pediatr Adolesc Med. 148:711, 1994

Santer DM, Michaelsen VE, Erkonen WE, et al. A comparison of educational interventions. Multimedia textbook, standard lecture, and printed textbook. Arch Pediatr Adolesc Med. 149:297, 1995

Satava R. Virtual reality surgical simulator: the first steps. Surg Endosc. 7:203, 1993

Schatz BR. Information retrieval in digital libraries: bringing search to the Net. Science. 275:327, 1997

Scherer WT, White CC, Wilson EC. UROGEN: An expert system for the diagnosis and treatment of female urogenital complaints. In Blum BI (ed): Proceedings of the 11th Annual Symposium on Computer Applications in Medical Care, p 189. Silver Spring, MD: IEEE Computer Society Press, 1987

Schilling J, Faisst K, Kapetanios E, Wyss P, Norrie MC, Gutzwiller F. Appropriateness and necessity research on the Internet: using a "second opinion system." Methods Inf Med. 39:233-7, 2000

Schneier B. Applied Cryptography, 2nd ed. New York: John Wiley & Sons, 1996

Sekikawa A, Sa ER, Acosta B, Aaron DJ, LaPorte RE. Internet mirror sites. Lancet. 355(9219):2000, 2000

Sherry E. Trauma and orthopaedic surgery on the Internet. J Bone Joint Surg Br. 81:558, 1999

Shortliffe EH. Computer-based clinical decision aids: Some practical considerations. In Lindberg DA, Collen MF, Van Brunt EE (eds): Proceedings of the AMIA Congress, 1982, p 295. New York: Masson, 1982

Shortliffe EH. Medical informatics meets medical education. JAMA. 273:1061, 1064, 1995

Skolnick AA. Protecting privacy of computerized patient information may lie in the cards. JAMA. 272:187, 1994

Small SL, Muechler EK. Heuristic determination of relevant diagnostic procedures in a medical expert system for gynecology. Am J Obstet Gynecol. 161:17, 1989

Smith A, Elkind A, Eardley A. Making cervical screening work. Br Med J Clin Res. 298:1662, 1989

Smith R. Computers in medicine: searching for the rainbow and the pot of gold. Br Med J. 284:1859, 1982

Smith RP, Holzman GB. The application of a computer database system to the generation of hospital discharge summaries. Obstet Gynecol. 73:803, 1989

Spielberg AR. On call and online: sociohistorical, legal, and ethical implications of e-mail for the patient-physician relationship. JAMA. 280:1353, 1998

Spooner SA. On-line resources for pediatricians. Arch Pediatr Adolesc Med. 149:1160, 1995

Stair TO, Howell JM. Effect on medical education of computerized physician order entry. Acad Med. 70:543, 1995

Steckner K, Borkowski R. On-line resources for the Pain Medicine physician. Reg Anesth Pain Med. 25:291-5, 2000

Strickland NH, Allison DJ, Gishen P. Technical note: a radiological education system—organization of an image library. Br J Radiol. 68:524, 1995

Strum S. Consultation and patient information on the Internet: the patients' forum. Br J Urol. 80 suppl 3:22, 1997

Suchard MA, Hadfield R, Elliott T, Kennedy S. Beyond providing information: the Internet as a research tool in reproductive medicine. Human Reprod. 13:6, 1998

Suzuki Y, Nakamura M. Internet in nuclear medicine. Ann Nuclear Med. 11:7, 1997

Tan JK, Hanna J. Integrating health care with information technology: knitting patient information through networking. Health Care Manage Rev. 19:72, 1994

Taylor KS. Patient software: consultation at the stroke of a key. Hosp Health Netw. 68:72, 1994

Ten Haken JD, Love SJ, Calhoun JG, et al. The integration of computer conferencing into the medical school curriculum. Med Teach. 11:213, 1989

Tierney WM, Miller ME, Overhage JM, McDonald CJ. Physician inpatient order writing on microcomputer workstations: effects on resource utilization. JAMA. 269:379, 1993

Tilson ER, Rodgers AT, Cross DS, Tanenbaum BG. Internet listservers in radiology. Radiol Technol. 69:267, 1998

Tiplady B, Crompton GK, Brackenridge D. Electronic diaries for asthma. Br Med J. 310:1469, 1995

Turner RC, Peden JG Jr, O'Brein K. Patient-carried card prompts vs computer-generated prompts to remind private practice patients to perform health maintenance measures. Arch Intern Med. 154:1957, 1994

Vale JA, Thompson AC. Information technology, the Internet and the urologist. Br J Urol. 80 (suppl 3):8, 1997

Van Hine P, Pearse WH. The IAMS project of the American College of Obstetricians and Gynecologists: using information technology to improve health care of women. Bull Med Libr Assoc. 76:237, 1988

Waldrop MM. On-line archives let biologists interrogate the genome. Science. 269:1356, 1995

Wang KK, Wong Kee Song LM. The physician and the Internet. Mayo Clin Proc. 72:66, 1997

Weaver J. Patient education: an innovative computer approach. Nurs Manage. 26:78, 1995

Webber WB, Summers AN, Rinehart GC. Computer-based multimedia in plastic surgery education. Plast Reconstr Surg. 93:1290, 1994

Wheeler LA, Wheeler ML, Ours P, et al. Use of CAAI/video in diabetes patient nutrition education. In Dayhoff R (ed): Proceedings of the 7th Annual Symposium on Computer Applications in Medical Care, p 961. Silver Spring, MD: IEEE Computer Society Press, 1983

Wilcke JR. Therapeutic information on the Internet. Vet Clin North Am [Small Anim Pract]. 28:449, 1998

Williams TG, Hirsch VJ, Stasburg E. The development of a gynecology data base collection system. Am J Perinatol. 2:259, 1985

Wofford MM, Wofford JL. The affordability and efficacy of MCAI. Arch Intern Med. 155:1682, 1995

Wood FB, Lyon B, Schell MB, Kitendaugh P, Cid VH, Siegel ER. Public library consumer health information pilot project: results of a National Library of Medicine evaluation. Bull Med Libr Assoc. 88:314-22, 2000

Woods SE, Coggan JM. Developing a medical informatics education program to support a statewide health information network. Bull Med Libr Assoc. 82:147, 1994

Yamamoto LG, Suh PJ. Accessing and using the Internet's World Wide Web for emergency physicians. Am J Emerg Med. 14:302, 1996

Zador IE, Sokol RJ. Ultrasound in cyberspace. Ultrasound Obstet Gynecol. 15:56-61, 2000

Zimmermann PR. Cryptography for the Internet. Sci Am. 279(4):110, 1998

Appendix 2
Health-Related Internet Resources

General Internet Guides

General Internet Guides

Medical Internet Guides

beWELL.com

Hosted by Blackwell Science publishers. Features highlighted topics, electronic magazines, news, and a diagnostic procedures resource.
World Wide Web URL: http://beWELL.com/

The Daily Apple

Medical health guide full of the news and advice. Find resources on illness, disease prevention, lifestyle, family, and everyday health.
World Wide Web URL: http://thedailyapple.com/

Doctor's Guide

A doctor's guide to the Internet resources that includes links, news, medical alerts, and list of conferences and meetings.
World Wide Web URL: http://www.pslgroup.com/MEDRES.HTM

Doctor's Guide to the Internet

Gives medical news and alerts, new drug advice, medical conference details, publications, and patient information and resources. Doctor's Guide was designed to help physicians cost-effectively harness the resources of the Internet and the World Wide Web.
World Wide Web URL: http://www.docguide.com/default.htm

The Doctors' Home Page

Numerous links to medical sites of interest, including patient education materials, medical quotes, medical humor, and others.
World Wide Web URL: http://www.DoctorsPage.net

Family Internet

Browse the health section for resources on medical conditions and family health or search the database for information.
World Wide Web URL: http://www.familyInternet.com/frames.html

Health on the Net

A search engine for finding medically related health sites on the Internet.
World Wide Web URL: http://www.hon.ch/

Healthtouch

Find up-to-date information on health, wellness, diseases, and illnesses. Topics include the prevention and treatment information on AIDS, allergy, asthma, dental health, diet and nutrition, drug and alcohol abuse, eye diseases, eating disorders, family planning, headaches, mental health, poison prevention, sexually transmitted diseases, and other health areas.
World Wide Web URL: http://www.healthtouch.com/level1/hi_toc.htm

Healthweb

HealthWeb provides links to specific, evaluated information resources on the World Wide Web selected by librarians and information professionals at leading academic medical centers in the Midwest. Selection emphasizes quality information aimed at assisting health care professionals as well as consumers in meeting their health information needs.
World Wide Web URL: http://healthweb.org/index.cfm

InteliHealth-Johns Hopkins

Features daily news articles, health quizzes, ask-the-doc, health library, and loads of informative health information.
World Wide Web URL: http://www.intellihealth.com/IH/ihtIH

Reuters Health Information Services

Cover the important news stories in health and medicine each business day. Stories are linked to a drug database with searchable news archive. Consumer information is free, professional information is by subscription.
World Wide Web URL: http://www.reutershealth.com/

The WWW Virtual Library: Biosciences: Medicine

A "virtual library" of Internet sites and resources.
World Wide Web URL: http://www.ohsu.edu/cliniweb/wwwvl/

Portals, Directories, and Guides (Free)

Achoo—On Line Health care Services

One of the greatest hurdles for the health care sector is the sheer volume of information available through the Internet. Achoo acts as a jump point and information resource for the medical community and all other Internet users interested in health care information. The comprehensive Internet health care directory contains over 7,400 links. Hundreds of health care-related Usenet discussions are archived here and current Headline News is provided. Achoo also offers an Internet health care directory with sites categorized by the human life, the practice of medicine, and the business of health.
World Wide Web URL: http://www.achoo.com/

Be Well

Formerly part of HealthGate, beWELL.com offers resource centers for numerous conditions and diseases (allergies, migraines, and breast cancer, among many others). The articles are accessible (sometimes verging on oversimplification) and make a useful starting point for the recently diagnosed. The site also includes a Diagnostic Procedures Handbook, which describes (in clinical detail) medical tests such as MRIs and CAT scans.
World Wide Web URL: http://www.bewell.com

Case Management Resource

Searchable guide of over 110,000 specialty health care services, facilities, businesses, programs, and organizations.
World Wide Web URL: http://www.cmrg.com/

Essential Links to Medicine

An extentsive list of on-line resources to medicine, medical information, facilities, diseases, education, libraries, organizations, news, newsgroups, newsletters, and other health-related matters.
World Wide Web URL: http://www.EL.com/elinks/medicine/

HandiLinks—Health Directory

Information guide indexed in an alphabetical format. Find resources on interesting and unusual topics including blood banks and bee pollen.
World Wide Web URL: http://www.ahandyguide.com/cat1/Health.htm

Health Canada Online

Health Canada is the federal department responsible for helping the people of Canada maintain and improve their health. This site offers news and information about health maintenance and specific diseases in either English or French. The site is searchable and contains lots of useful facts such as information for travelers, food guides, and news stories.
World Wide Web URL: http://www.hc-sc.gc.ca/english/

Health Oasis / Mayo Clinic Health Guide

Health and medical news geared to patients as well as the general public, including daily news on new drugs and treatments. Includes a database of heart-healthy recipes, the best men's health center on the Web, and a library of articles answering commonly asked health questions ranging from diabetes risk to the long-term effects of cracking your knuckles.
World Wide Web URL: http://www.mayohealth.org/home

HealthAnswers

Search for particular illness using the keyword and phrase search facility. Contains health news, tips, health and travel info, and a quiz.
World Wide Web URL: http://www.healthanswers.com/default.asp

HealthAtoZ

HealthAtoZ allows users to search for a health topic or find health sites within its directory. Each topic may contain information from or link to several hundred sites.
World Wide Web URL: http://www.healthatoz.com

Healthfinder

Developed by the U.S. Department of Health and Human Services, this is an excellent gateway Web site that links to a broad range of consumer health and human services information resources produced by the federal government and its many partner organizations.
World Wide Web URL: http://www.healthfinder.org

Healthy.Net Home Page—HealthWorld Online

With a strong emphasis on alternative and complementary therapies, Health-World Online provides a variety of resources on issues including nutrition,

fitness, and self-care. The interface is an nice graphic representation of a small town.
World Wide Web URL: http://www.healthy.net/

Medical Matrix

Excellent source of medically related Web sites each with a brief description. Requires registration or a browser that allow cookies.
World Wide Web URL: http://www.medmatrix.org/index.asp

MedicineNet

Developed and maintained by physicians, MedicineNet provides a good A-to-Z reference outlining the symptoms and treatment of various diseases. But hypochondriacs beware: like doctors with a clumsy bedside manner, the articles tend to ask as many questions as they answer. (Your head hurts? It's probably a migraine. Unless it's a brain tumor.)
World Wide Web URL: http://www.medicinenet.com/Script/Main/hp.asp

Medscape

Medscape for health professionals and interested consumers, features thousands of full-text, peer-reviewed articles, medical news, Medline, and interactive quizzes.
World Wide Web URL: http://www.medscape.com/default.mhtml

Medsite

Medsite is a medical search engine linked to more than 10,000 reviewed medical sites. There are direct links to Medline and Daily Medical News, as well as access to on-line chatrooms. This commercial site can lead to almost anywhere in the Web health world.
World Wide Web URL: http://www.medSite.com/

MedWeb: Biomedical Internet Resources

Maintained by Emory University Health Sciences Center Library, this site offers links to other medical information sites and resources.
World Wide Web URL: http://www.MedWeb.Emory.Edu/MedWeb/

The National Institutes of Health

This is the portal for the National Institutes of Health. It provides information about resources available through the NIH, with appropriate links.
World Wide Web URL: http://www.nih.gov/

National Women's Health Resource Center

Quite possibly the leading U.S. federal clearinghouse for women's health information.
World Wide Web URL: http://www.healthywomen.org/

New York Online Access to Health

Patient oriented and hosted by the New York Online Access to Health. Vast resource with loads of information on health and diseases organized by topic or search.
World Wide Web URL: http://www.noah-health.org/

Primary Care Internet Guide

This site has an extensive list of indexed resources. Maintained by the University of Bergen, Norway.
World Wide Web URL: http://www.uib.no/isf/guide/guide.htm

Virtual Hospital

Presented by the Electric Differential Multimedia Laboratory, Department of Radiology, University of Iowa College of Medicine, Iowa City, Iowa. This site includes information for patients and providers, including textbooks, articles, images, and links.
World Wide Web URL: http://vh.org/

Virtual Naval Hopsital

Presented by the Electric Differential Multimedia Laboratory, Department of Radiology, University of Iowa College of Medicine, Iowa City, Iowa. Library of authoritative medical info covering health issues pertinent to naval service. Includes safety, drug issues, dental, and diseases.
World Wide Web URL: http://www.vnh.org/

Wheeless' Textbook of Orthopaedics

Site with links of interest to both orthopedists and primary care physicians who use the Internet.
World Wide Web URL: http://www.medmedia.com/

The Wonderful Worlds of Internal Medicine and Pediatrics

A series of links and list dealing with issues revolving around internal medicine and pediatrics individually and as a combined specialty.
World Wide Web URL: http://ourworld.compuserve.com/homepages/anduril/medicin2.htm

Yahoo Alternative Medicine Guide

A link to alternative medicine sites on the Web. Includes acupuncture, homeopathy, naturopathy, music therapy, and others.
World Wide Web URL: http://www.yahoo.com/Health/Alternative_Medicine/

Portals, Directories, and Guides (Subscription)

HealthGate Biomedical Databases

Includes CME, biomedical databases, literature searches, etc. Free and fee-based services available.
World Wide Web URL: http://www.healthgate.com

HealthGate Medline

Free search of the medical journal abstract database. Additional services available for a fee.
World Wide Web URL: http://www3.healthgate.com

HealthWorld Medline

Searching and retrieval of citations and abstracts at no charge. Full document delivery for a fee.
World Wide Web URL: http://www.healthy.net/library/search/medline.htm

Paper Chase Medical Literature Searching

A fee-based system that allows searches of Medline, Cancerlit, AIDSline, and other large medical publication archives.
World Wide Web URL: http://www.paperchase.com

Medline and Other Information Providers

Dr. Felix's Free Medline Page

Links to Web sites where you can search Medline for free.
World Wide Web URL: http://www.beaker.iupui.edu/drfelix/

The US National Library of Medicine

Entry point for the National Library of Medicine including general information, databases, and photographic archives. Connections to comprehensive databases of medical information such as MEDLARS and MEDLINE are also available.
World Wide Web URL: http://www.nlm.nih.gov/

Medical News and Information

Alliance for Health Reform

The Alliance for Health Reform is a nonpartisan organization that conducts research on a variety of health care issues, including children's health, Medicare, and the cost and availability of health care. Provides objective information in a number of formats to journalists, elected officials and their staffs, and other shapers of public opinion.
World Wide Web URL: http://www.allhealth.org

InteliHealth

Maintained by Johns Hopkins Health Information Services, this site provides general health news and information along with disease-specific updates. Offers drug indexes, ask-a-doc, and self-assessment features.
World Wide Web URL: http://www.intelihealth.com/IH/ihtIH

On Health

A site that presents a wide-ranging and ever-changing selection of medical topics geared for the general public. The information is current and dependable

and may be searched by topic or even by items of local interest. By setting cookies it allows the user to create a personal place for searching and saving information that's important to the individual. It searches a carefully selected universe of trustworthy health and medical resources on the Web on a daily basis and lets the user know when something new is found.
World Wide Web URL: http://www.mywebmd.com

QuackWatch

Quackwatch, Inc., a member of Consumer Federation of America, is a nonprofit corporation whose purpose is to combat health-related frauds, myths, fads, and fallacies. Founded by Dr. Stephen Barrett in 1969 as the Lehigh Valley Committee Against Health Fraud, it was incorporated in 1970 and assumed its current name in 1997. The information provided is also available in French and German.
World Wide Web URL: http://www.quackwatch.com/

Medical Internet Guides

Computers in Medicine—Starter Bookmarks

The purpose of these bookmarks is to introduce the user to some of the different types of medically useful sites on the Internet. It is hoped that the list will serve as a useful starting point for those just beginning to explore the Internet and will introduce those with more experience to types of sites with which they might not have been familiar.
World Wide Web URL: http://www.acponline.org/computer/ccp/ bookmark/

Computers in Medicine—Web Watch

Web Sites for Internists is the internist's guide to medical resources on the Internet. It is intended to be selective, rather than comprehensive, to save the user from having to wade through extensive lists.
World Wide Web URL: http://www.acponline.org/computer/ccp/ bookmark/index.html

Healthtouch

The site provides a long list of links to health-related sites, both public and private.
World Wide Web URL: http://www.healthtouch.com

Kindly Doctor Knows Health and Medicine Site

Kindly Doctor Knows Health and Medicine Site is an effort to gather related sites from the World Wide Web and present them in such a way that both doctor and patient will find them convenient.
World Wide Web URL: http://members.tripod.com/~Terry222/index.html

MedPedia

A personal set of links to medically related sites designed for patients and physicians alike.
World Wide Web URL: http://www.evansville.net/~wbbebout/

Physician's Guide to the Internet

A general portal to continuing education opportunities.
World Wide Web URL: http://physiciansguide.com/educ.html

Search for Medical Information

Aimed at consumers, this site offers step-by-step instructions for finding medical information in medical libraries and organizations on the Web.
World Wide Web URL: http://204.17.98.73/midlib/www.htm

Medline and Other Information Providers

BioMedNet.com

BioMedNet.com offers registered users access to print journals, but in some cases there is a fee for downloading the articles that varies from $2.50 to $25.00.
World Wide Web URL: http://www.bmn.com

British Medical Association

The BMA provides free and unlimited access to Medline and EMBASE, but only to members of the association. To use this service, you need a USERID and a PASSWORD.
World Wide Web URL: http://ovid.bma.org.uk/

Epocrates

This is the site of a supplier of clinical information modules for portable Palm (and Palm compatible) computers. Its main offering is a drug dosing and usage database than can be easily downloaded and installed on your computer.
World Wide Web URL: http://www.epocrates.com

InteliHealth

A collaboration of Harvard Medical School and the InteliHealth corporation, this site provides consumer information, personalized e-mails on health topics, and a commercial side that sells health-related products and services.
World Wide Web URL: http://www.intelihealth.com

Journal Watch Online

Browse and search Journal Watch. Twice-weekly on-line summaries of new medical research.
World Wide Web URL: http://www.jwatch.org/

Medicine OnLine

Medicine OnLine is published by UltiTech, Inc. of Stratford, CT, and offers medical information and education in oncology and HIV/AIDS, Medline literature searches, Daily Medical News, Cancer Forums discussion groups, and reports from medical meetings for health care professionals, patients, and other interested consumers.
World Wide Web URL: http://www.meds.com

Medis Medi-Search

A search facility that indexes abstracts and articles from major medical journals. Search results return links back to the original article, including URL locations.
World Wide Web URL: http://www.docnet.org.uk/medis/search-old.html

Medline Database at Community of Science, Inc

The mission of the Community of Science (COS) is to provide rapid, easy-to-use information about scientists and the funding of science. The Community of Science is a global registry designed to provide accurate, timely, easy-to-access information about what new funding opportunities exist, and who is working on what subject and where. This site permits searches of the entire Medline

database, new entries, or abstracts in specific journals. Free and fee subscriptions available.
World Wide Web URL: http://www.cos.com

Medscape Medline Search

Presents a Medline search that is coupled with a search of Medscape's full-text articles. Requires membership (which is free).
World Wide Web URL: http://www.medscape.com/misc/
FormMedlineInfLive.html

National Cancer Institute

News and abstracts from the *Journal of the National Cancer Institute* (JNCI) and other NCI publications. Connect with CANCERLIT, a comprehensive archival file of more than 1,000,000 bibliographic records describing cancer results published for the past 30 years in biomedical journals, proceedings of scientific meetings, books, technical reports, and other documents.
World Wide Web URL: http://wwicic.nci.nih.gov

Ovid On Call Medline and Medical Databases

An on-line interface for searches of Medline, AIDSline, and 15 top medical journals. Presents full-text articles and abstracts. Includes charts, photographs, and graphics.
World Wide Web URL: http://preview.ovid.com/sales/medical.cfm

Topicdoc

A fast, user-friendly, topic-driven medical literature service offering peer-reviewed articles from the National Library of Medicine. TopicDoc facilitates getting medical information for an array of selected topics without the necessity of medical research training or access to a medical library. You can maintain your own list of personal topics and have the option to receive e-mail notification when a new listing is posted.
World Wide Web URL: http://www.topicdoc.com

Continuing Education

Academia Medica Home Page

Catalog and home page for Academia Medica, producers of high-quality interactive multimedia CME programs for physicians.
World Wide Web URL: http://www.acad-med.co.il/

Cme-ce.com

This site provides CME and CE credited learning activities to doctors, nurses, pharmacists, and allied health professionals. The site includes free access a physician referral database, health care links, on-line registration to symposia, medical teleconferences, etc., as well as a bookstore and free offer section. The accredited activities on CME-CE.COM are a free service supported by unrestricted educational grants. A quick, one-time registration is required to ensure proper awarding of continuing education credits.
World Wide Web URL: http://www.cme-ce.com/

CMEWeb Medical Education for Physicians

Emergency medicine and primary care tests for physicians with on-line registration and certificates.
World Wide Web URL: http://www.cmeweb.com

Cyber University

CyberUniversity.net is a portal for comprehensive medical education for the physician and other health care professionals. It offers preparatory exams for undergraduate, graduate, and postgraduate medical education. This includes preparation for specialty board certification and medical licensing. Cyber University also offers a wide range of continuing medical education (CME) courses. It provides education for physician practice management, and medical research.
World Wide Web URL: http://www.cyberuniversity.net/Home.asp

The Emergency Medicine and Primary Care Home Page

This site provides educational resources for emergency and primary care physicians and health care providers.
World Wide Web URL: http://www.embbs.com/

Health care Education and Learning Information Exchange

Helix (Health care Education Learning and Information Exchange) is a meta-health care site on the World Wide Web offering professional education and information for all health practitioners and their patients. Sponsored and managed by the Glaxo Wellcome Health care Education Department, HELIX on the World Wide Web offers point-and-click access to a wealth of health information on the Internet as well as the Web sites of a number of state and national medical, pharmacy, and nursing associations. Membership is free via on-line registration. This site also offers Medline access.
World Wide Web URL: http://www.HELIX.com

Internet Medical Education, Inc.

This site offers both physician and consumer medical education including reviews, quizzes, and an expert system for the 12-lead ECG and for cardiac rhythm analysis.
World Wide Web URL: http://www.med-edu.com/index.html

MDChoice.com

A site offering access to several types of continuing education and peer-reviewed content. The site also offers searchable content that varies from chapters to news articles.
World Wide Web URL: http://www.mdchoice.com/

Medical Education Online (MEO)

Medical Education Online (MEO) is a forum for disseminating information on educating physicians and other health professionals. Manuscripts on any aspect of the process of training health professionals are considered for peer-reviewed publication in their electronic journal. In addition to manuscripts, MEO provides a repository for resources such as curricula, data sets, syllabi, software, and instructional material developers wish to make available to the health education community. The site also posts informational messages and links to World Wide Web sites of interest to health science educators.
World Wide Web URL: http://www.med-ed-online.org

New Hampshire MedNet

Developed by the New Hampshire Medical Society, the New Hampshire Med Net facilitates access to a variety of resources for medical providers in the region. Many new Internet-based communication and education initiatives are under development at this site.
World Wide Web URL: http://www.nhmednet.org/default.htm

Physicians' News Digest

A comprehensive database of continuing medical education programs searchable by topic, date, sponsor, and location.
World Wide Web URL: http://www.physiciansnews.com/cme.html

PubMed

NLM's search service to access the 9 million citations in MEDLINE and Pre-MEDLINE (with links to participating on-line journals), and other related databases.
World Wide Web URL: http://www.ncbi.nlm.nih.gov/PubMed/

Practice Management or Marketing

Clinical Multimedia Laboratory

The Clinical Multimedia Laboratory at the University of Pittsburgh Medical Center hosts this site that contains information about the integration of clinical images into an electronic medical record system.
World Wide Web URL: http://www.cml.upmc.edu/

General

Association of American Medical Colleges

The medical schools and programs are listed alphabetically in order of state or province. It is also indicated whether each school participates in the American Medical College Application Service (AMCAS), the University of Texas System Medical and Dental Application Center (UTSMDAC), or the Ontario Medical School Application Service (OMSAS).
World Wide Web URL: http://www.aamc.org

Clinical Medical Education at Kansas

Contains materials designed to enhance medical education in cardiology, radiology, dermatology, and hematology.
World Wide Web URL: http://www.kumc.edu

CME Software Reviews

Brief reviews of medical education software.
World Wide Web URL: http://www.webcom.com/~wooming/mededuc.html

The Cochrane Collaboration

The Cochrane Collaboration has developed in response to Dr. Cochrane's call for systematic, up-to-date reviews of all relevant randomized clinical trials of health care. Cochrane's suggestion that the methods used to prepare and maintain reviews of controlled trials in pregnancy and childbirth should be applied more widely was taken up by the Research and Development Programme, initiated to support the United Kingdom's National Health Service. Funds were provided to establish a "Cochrane Centre," to collaborate with others, in the UK and elsewhere, to facilitate systematic reviews of randomized controlled trials across all areas of health care. This site provides access to this information.

World Wide Web URL: http://hiru.mcmaster.ca/cochrane/

Go Ask Alice

A consumer-oriented collection of over 1,000 questions and answers in a searchable format. Geared toward college students and teenagers, Go Ask Alice offers practical, nonjudgmental responses to common questions about relationships, sexuality, drugs, and other mysteries that are hard to ask about and even harder to answer.

World Wide Web URL: http://www.goaskalice.columbia.edu/

Grateful Med

Access point to the National Library of Medicine site. This site has a search engine that allows retrieval of relevant articles and citations. Requires a National Library of Medicine on-line account.

World Wide Web URL: http://igm.nlm.nih.gov/

Medical Education Online

Articles, curriculum outlines, data sets, interactive discussion forums, cases, and software that cover health professional training and problem-based learning. Provided by the University of Texas Medical Branch at Galveston.

World Wide Web URL: http://www.med-ed-online.org/

The Residency Page

Lists all known medical residencies.

World Wide Web URL: http://www.residencysite.com

ScHARR—Netting the Evidence

An Internet site that is devoted to applying research data to develop evidence-based medical practice is supplied by the School of Health and Related Research (ScHARR), in Sheffield, UK. ScHARR is one of the four schools in the faculty of medicine at the University of Sheffield. It is a significant university-based

concentration of health-related information in Trent and one of the most important in the UK.
World Wide Web URL: http://www.shef.ac.uk/~scharr/ir/netting/

Stanford MedWorld

This is the independent student site sponsored by the Stanford Medical Alumni Association. The site provides world-wide medical student articles and Internet links that enhance the medical training process.
World Wide Web URL: http://medworld.stanford.edu/home/

Webrounds at Williams and Wilkins

An interactive, on-line journal for medical students that permits users to browse professional journal articles and abstracts and learn about residency programs.
World Wide Web URL: http://www.wwilkins.com/rounds/index.html

Indexes

Achoo Health care Online—Reference sources

Achoo maintains an extensive set of links to various journals.
World Wide Web URL: http://www.achoo.com/features/refsources/
default.asp

CertiFacts Online

This site is sponsored by the American Board of Medical Specialties (ABMS) and operated by TMPW, Inc. The site is a primary source verification of the board certification status of medical specialists in all ABMS recognized specialties and subspecialties. You can obtain password-protected access to ABMS data of board certification information on over 500,000 physicians, with effective and expiration dates displayed. (It does require the correct spelling of the physician's name.) This is primarily used by credentialing committees and similar bodies.
World Wide Web URL: http://www.certifacts.org

The Doctor Directory

A database of over 500,000 doctors and physicians nationwide. Find a physician by city or state, and get a location map to to guide you.
World Wide Web URL: http://www.doctordirectory.com/Doctors/
Directory/Default.asp?Reference=DrDir.PhysicianStates&TargetPage=
Details.asp

Human GenomeBrowser

The ultimate index site is the Human Genome Browser hosted by the University of California, Santa Cruz. This site begins with a search box for you to enter the gene ID number, position, or key word. Results are displayed as a rulerlike box loaded with information about that region of the human genome.
World Wide Web URL: http://genome.ucsc.edu/goldenPath/hgTracks.html

Instructions to Authors in the Health Sciences

This site is maintained by the Raymon H. Mulford library at the Medical College of Ohio and is invaluable as a resource for anyone wishing to publish in a medical journal. The site has links to specific information for authors and submission requirements, but also links to information needed for medical research and publishing in general.
World Wide Web URL: http://www.mco.edu/lib/instr/libinsta.html

Medical World Search

Medical World Search is best used for specific clinical searches involving diseases and conditions. The site allows you to search the full text of nearly 100,000 Web pages from thousands of medical sites.
World Wide Web URL: http://www.mwsearch.com

Medsite

Medsite is a medical search engine linked to more than 10,000 reviewed medical sites. There are direct links to Medline and Daily Medical News, as well as access to on-line chatrooms. This commercial site can lead to almost anywhere in the Web health world.
World Wide Web URL: http://www.medSite.com/

MedWeb Educational Resources

Well-maintained links to guides, sites, journals, organizations, and documents for a general audience.
World Wide Web URL: http://www.medweb.emory.edu/MedWeb/

NCI CANCERNET Database—National Cancer Institute

CancerNet from the National Cancer Institute (NCI) provides up-to-date information for cancer patients as well as physicians. In addition to concise summaries about prognosis, staging, and treatment for more than 80 tumor types, information about drugs, supportive care, screening, prevention, and

selected clinical trials can be found. This redistribution is maintained by the University of Bonn.
World Wide Web URL: http://imsdd.meb.uni-bonn.de/cancernet/ cancernet.html

Office of Medical Informatics Education at Johns Hopkins

Global links that enable students to access course information, lecture notes, handouts, and sample exams in a searchable, lecture-by-lecture format.
World Wide Web URL: http://omie.med.jhmi.edu/

WebMedLit

Currently tracking 18 medical journals. View the latest medical literature on the Web by topic including AIDS/virology, cardiology, cancer/oncology, dermatology, diabetes/endocrinology, gastroenterology, medical economics, neurology and women's health.
World Wide Web URL: http://www.webmedlit.com/

Sites

Cancer Control Journal On-line CME

CME credits are offered for reading issues and answering the questions posed in the posttest.
World Wide Web URL: http://moffitt.usf.edu/pubs/ccj/

Clinical Concepts CME Home Study Courses

The Southern Medical Association maintains this fee-based continuing education site. Deals with various patient care topics.
World Wide Web URL: http://www.sma.org/education/index.htm

Clinical Laboratory Improvement Act On-line CME Course

Provides credit hours needed for physicians to be lab directors under CLIA.
World Wide Web URL: http://vh.radiology.uiowa.edu/Providers/CME/ CLIA/CLIAHP.html

Emergency Medical Abstracts On-line

Emergency physicians can obtain CME credits at this site.
World Wide Web URL: http://ccme.org

Medconnect Interactive Education Cases

Accredited for CME by the American College of Emergency Physicians, this site has "Cases of the Month" to sharpen skills.
World Wide Web URL: http://www.medconnect.com/home-cas.htm

Southern Medical Association

The Southern Medical Association maintains a fee-based (free for members) continuing education site that can easily be reached from the navigation tools on the left side of the frame.
World Wide Web URL: http://www.sma.org

University of Michigan Medical Center

Educational resources including a thoracic radiology tutorial and a medical software catalog.
World Wide Web URL: http://www.med.umich.edu/lrc/

University of Washington CME Teaching Files

This site has radiology and anatomy teaching files. CME credit is available.
World Wide Web URL: http://www.rad.washington.edu

WebPath Pathology Images CME

The University of Utah provides this CME opportunity. Images on various topics including AIDS and bone pathology.
World Wide Web URL: http://medstat.med.utah.edu/WebPath/ webpath.html#MENU

Meetings

Academic Medicine Events and Meetings

A list from the Association of American Medical Colleges.
World Wide Web URL: http://www.aamc.org/meetings/start.htm

AMA On-line CME Locator

A quick access point to U.S. continuing medical education accreditied AMA category I CME providers and activities. Search criteria include the type of

CME activity, disease subject area, location by a map of states, dates, faculty, and titles.
World Wide Web URL: http://www.ama-assn.org/cgi-bin/cme-redir

CMESearch Continuing Medical Education Courses

A database searchable by location, date, specialty, and profession. This site also allows on-line registration and travel arrangements to be made.
World Wide Web URL: http://www.cmesearch.com/

Doctors' Guide to the Internet Medical Meetings

A comprehensive searchable list of medical meetings and conferences organized by catagory is available through this site.
World Wide Web URL: http://www.pslgroup.com/MEDSITES.HTM

Events in Bioscience and Medicine

Meetings and workshops for bioscientists and clinicians. All meetings are ordered by date and subject (includes biochemistry, biotechnology, cancer research, cardiovascular research, cell and molecular biology, gene therapy, genetics, molecular diagnostics, neurology/neuroscience).
World Wide Web URL: http://www.hum-molgen.de/meetings/index.php3

Forums

DermDigest—The On-line Dermatology Conference

Information, on-line interactions, skin care tips, and regular columns make up this interesting site.
World Wide Web URL: http://dermdigest.com/

Medical Journal Club on the Web

An on-line, interactive general medical "journal club" that summarizes internal medicine articles from the recent medical literature and appends reader comments.
World Wide Web URL: http://www.webcom.com/mjljweb/jrnlclb/index.html

Cases

Adult Echocardiography @Columbia-Presbyterian Medical Center

This site offers a series of images in echocardiography. Two formats are available to view images. A question and answer method allows physicians and ultrasound technologists to test themselves. The library allows the individual to view images based on the diagnosis.
World Wide Web URL: http://cpmcnet.columbia.edu:80/dept/cardiology/echo/

Albert Einstein Multimedia Modules

Multimedia medical school curriculum is hosted at this site.
World Wide Web URL: http://cobweb.aecom.yu.edu/

Digital Image Gallery

Over 300 3D anatomy clipart and 100 AVI animations rendered from the best selection of 3D anatomy models. This low-cost collection is perfect for students and project developers. Commercial license available.
World Wide Web URL: http://www.posturepro.com/digit.htm

Interactive Colorado Medical Rounds

The University of Colorado provides these care studies and discussions.
World Wide Web URL: http://www.uchsc.edu/sm/pmb/medrounds/index.html

The Interactive Patient

Marshall University maintains a WWW interactive medical education tool that simulates a patient encounter. The user asks history questions, performs a physical examination, orders tests, and submits a diagnosis and treatment plan. Detailed feedback is provided.
World Wide Web URL: http://medicus.marshall.edu/medicus.htm

Lyola University Medical Education Network

Hypertext medical educational resources in anatomy, histology, pathology, and other fields presented with graphics and text.
World Wide Web URL: http://www.meddean.luc.edu/lumen/

MedRounds Case Discussions at Colorado

This site allows users to enter, edit, and moderate case discussions.
**World Wide Web URL: http://www.uchsc.edu/sm/pmb/medrounds/
malindex.html**

Patient Simulations at the Virtual Hospital

An index of patient simulation case studies.
**World Wide Web URL: http://indy.radiology.uiowa.edu/Providers/
Simulations/PatientSimulations.html**

Pittsburgh Case Index by Patient History

A list of cases by patient diagnosis that presents examples of diseases, their
clinical hallmarks, and gross and microscopic markers. Continuing education
credits are available.
World Wide Web URL: http://path.upmc.edu:80/cme/index.htm

On-line journals

AMA Archives of Dermatology

The site offers information about the *Archives of Dermatology*, an opportunity to
register to get the table of contents via e-mail, and current or past tables of
contents.
World Wide Web URL: http://archderm.ama-assn.org/

The Annals of Thoracic Surgery

An on-line full text and graphics version (including video clips) of the *Annals of
Thoracic Surgery*.
World Wide Web URL: http://www.sts.org/annals/

British Medical Journal

This was one of the first major journals to post full text and archived articles.
World Wide Web URL: http://www.bmj.com

Canadian Journal of Plastic Surgery

This peer-reviewed journal contains case reports, papers, and articles related to the medical specialty of plastic surgery. This site offers the ability to search or view specific issues, including text and photographs.
World Wide Web URL: http://www.pulsus.com/plastics/home.htm

Canadian Medical Association Journal

Abstracts from Canada's premier peer-reviewed journal.
World Wide Web URL: http://www.cma.ca/cmaj/index.asp

Canadian Medical Association Journal Index

There are links to more than a dozen journals, newsletters, and reports from the Canadian Medical Association at this site maintained by the CMA.
World Wide Web URL: http://www.cma.ca/publications/index.htm

CDC Emerging Infectious Disease Journal

The journal *Emerging Infectious Diseases*, published by the National Center for Infectious Diseases, Centers for Disease Control and Prevention, tracks trends and provides synthesis and analysis of new and reemerging infectious disease issues around the world. The publisher welcomes articles from all disciplines whose study elucidates the factors influencing the emergence and reemergence of infectious diseases.
World Wide Web URL: http://www.cdc.gov/ncidod/eid/index.htm

Dermatology Online Journal

Visit this site for recent articles, proceedings, and announcements regarding dermatology.
World Wide Web URL: http://dermatology.cdlib.org/DOJvol1num1/ journal.html

Dermatology Times

A newspaper-format publication for the field of dermatology.
World Wide Web URL: http://www.dermatologytimes.com/

Digital Journal of Urology

An independent peer-reviewed medical journal of adult and pediatric urology. Features original articles, case presentations, meeting announcements, and patient information.
World Wide Web URL: http://www.duj.com/

Digital Urology Journal

A peer-reviewed journal of adult and pediatric urology on the World Wide Web.
World Wide Web URL: http://www.duj.com/

General Practice On-line

The *International Journal of General Practice and Primary Care.*
World Wide Web URL: http://www.priory.com/gp.htm

Geriatrics

Access to the journal *Geriatrics* is available at this site.
World Wide Web URL: http://www.geri.com/

Infection Control and Hospital Epidemiology

Infection Control and Hospital Epidemiology, the official journal of the Society for Health care Epidemiology of America, is a leading monthly journal providing original, peer-reviewed scientific articles for anyone involved with an infection control or epidemiology program with a hospital or health care facility.
World Wide Web URL: http://www.slackinc.com/general/iche/ichehome.htm

The International Journal of Psychiatry

On-line version of the *International Journal of Psychiatry.*
World Wide Web URL: http://psychiatry.mc.duke.edu/ijpm/

JAMA Home Page—Americal Medical Association

Searchable article and abstract collection from JAMA. Requires registration.
World Wide Web URL: http://jama.ama-assn.org/

Journal of the American Academy of Dermatology

Information and news regarding dermatology and the AAD.
**World Wide Web URL: http://www.harcourthealth.com/scripts/om.dll/
serve?action=searchDB&searchDBfor=home&id=JD**

Journal of the American Academy of Orthopaedic Surgeons

This site offers the ability to search and view the table of contents from past
issues. Information about the journal and subscriptions are offered as well.
World Wide Web URL: http://www.JAAOS.ORG

The Journal of Bone and Joint Surgery (American Edition)

This site provides access to contents, abstracts, and subscription information.
World Wide Web URL: http://www.jbjs.org

Journal Watch Online

Browse and search Journal Watch. Twice-weekly on-line summaries of new
medical research.
World Wide Web URL: http://www.jwatch.org/

The Lancet

Offers full text summaries of selected articles from the *Lancet*.
World Wide Web URL: http://www.thelancet.com

Medical Journal of Australia

Peer-reviewed general and research articles. This site is unusual in that visitors
may post commentaries and contribute to the peer-review process prior to hard-
copy publication.
World Wide Web URL: http://www.library.usyd.edu.au/MJA/

National Cancer Institute

News and abstracts from the *Journal of the National Cancer Institute* (JNCI)
and other NCI publications. Connect with CANCERLIT, a comprehensive archival file of more than 1,000,000 bibliographic records describing cancer
results published for the past 30 years in biomedical journals, proceedings of
scientific meetings, books, technical reports, and other documents.
World Wide Web URL: http://www.nci.nih.gov

New England Journal of Medicine On-line

Extended abstracts and limited full text from the *New England Journal*.
World Wide Web URL: http://www.nejm.org/content/index.asp

Ophthalmology Times

Ophthalmology Times is a "physician-driven publication that disseminates news and information of a clinical, socioeconomic, and political nature in a timely and accurate manner for members of the ophthalmic community." This site connects you to the publisher.
World Wide Web URL: http://www.ophthalmologytimes.com/

Prevention Magazine

Not exactly a journal, this is the on-line version of the popular magazine.
World Wide Web URL: http://www.prevention.com/

ScripWorld Pharmaceutical News

Scrip is the only international, twice-weekly newsletter reporting on the pharmaceutical sector, covering prescription and OTC medicines and biotechnology news.
World Wide Web URL: http://www.pjbpubs.co.uk/scrip

Society for Endocrinology

The full text of articles published in *Endocrine-Related Cancer* is available freely to all. The full text of articles published in *Journal of Endocrinology* and *Journal of Molecular Endocrinology* is available free to institutions that subscribe to the printed version.
World Wide Web URL: http://journals.endocrinology.org/index.htm

Southern Medical Journal

Southern Medical Journal is a multispecialty publication distributed monthly to members. Southern Medical Association is testing the SMJ for future full Internet publication in addition to its current printed format. Starting with the June 1996 issue, the association placed these full-text journals on-line and will be adding all photos, tables, and advertising prior to official release.
World Wide Web URL: http://www.sma.org/smj/

Vascular Medicine

This site provides information about the journal *Vascular Medicine*. You can request a sample copy, subscribe, or review the instructions for authors.
World Wide Web URL: http://www.arnoldpublishers.com/Journals/ Journpages/1358863x.htm

WebMedLit

This site provides efficient access to the best medical journals on the Web. This site currently tracks 18 medical journals, and allows you to view the latest medical literature on the Web by topic. This site is a service of Web Medical Literature Services.
World Wide Web URL: http://www.webmedlit.com/

Medical Publishers

Audio Digest Foundation

The Audio Digest Foundation has provided medical professionals throughout the world with continuing medical education on audio tape since 1954. Its Web site offers a chance to view current topics and place orders.
World Wide Web URL: http://www.audio-digest.org/

Blackwell North America Core Publisher List

Based on entries in the Blackwell Approval Publishers List and supplemented by *Literary Market Place* and the Association of American University Presses Directory.
World Wide Web URL: http://www.blackwell.com/shelf/tools/cormed.htm

Centers for Disease Control and Prevention Publications

While the CDC is not in the medical publishing business, it does make available a wide variety of useful publications. This site provides a listing of its publications, software, and other products.
World Wide Web URL: http://www.cdc.gov/publications.htm

Krames Communications

Publisher of consumer-oriented information on medical, wellness, and injury prevention topics.
World Wide Web URL: http://www.krames.com

Lippincott Williams & Wilkins Publishers

Contains information about books, electronic media, and periodicals. The site offers a search engine and on-line ordering capabilities as well.
World Wide Web URL: http://www.wwilkins.com/

Medical Association Communications

Publisher for medical associations, meeting highlights, on-line medical journals. The site provides medical professionals with highlights from annual meetings of a number of medical associations, and selected continuing education programs in print and CD-ROM. Excerpts of full proceedings can be downloaded, or the original document or disk can be ordered at no cost.
World Wide Web URL: http://www.macmcm.com/

Mosby Publishing

"Mosby is the world's leading publisher of books, journals, and serial publications in the health sciences—medicine, nursing, allied health sciences, dentistry, veterinary medicine—and selected college disciplines—health, physical education and recreation, nutrition, and chemistry." Its WWW page has What's New at Mosby this month, a large catalog of health-sciences texts, videos, and software, and information about conferences and seminars that are currently being offered.
World Wide Web URL: http://www.harcourthealth.com/Mosby/index.html

Perimed Compliance Corp.

This corporation provides informed consent documents via the Internet. Requires a subscription.
World Wide Web URL: http://www.perimedusa.com/

Springer-Verlag

A searchable catalog of information and publications in the fields of biology and biomedicine, chemistry, computer science, economics and law, engineering, ecology and environmental sciences, geoscience, mathematics, medicine, physics and astronomy, psychology, and statistics.
World Wide Web URL: http://www.springer-ny.com/

Medical News and Information

AMA Physician Select: On-line Physician Finder

AMA Physician Select provides information on virtually every licensed physician in the United States and its possessions, including more than 650,000 doctors of medicine (MD) and doctors of osteopathy or osteopathic medicine (DO). All physician credential data have been verified for accuracy and authenticated by accrediting agencies, medical schools, residency training programs, licensing and certifying boards, and other data sources.
World Wide Web URL: http://www.ama-assn.org/aps/amahg.htm

AMA Science News Daily

Science news updates and materials from JAMA and other sources.
World Wide Web URL: http://www.ama-assn.org/sci-pubs/sci-news/1998/ pres_rel.htm

American Dental Association

Easy-to-read educational material for consumers combined with dental news, and a products and services guide.
World Wide Web URL: http://www.ada.org

American Medical News

Full-text version of the American Medical Association's publication covering professional, social, economic, and policy issues in medicine.
World Wide Web URL: http://www.ama-assn.org/public/journals/ amnews/amnews.htm

Centers for Disease Control and Prevention

This is the entry point for the CDC Web pages.
World Wide Web URL: http://www.cdc.gov

Health Care Financing Administration

The home page for the Health Care Financing Administration.
World Wide Web URL: http://www.hcfa.gov/

Health and Human Services

Access point for information about and from the Department of Health and Human Services.
World Wide Web URL: http://www.os.dhhs.gov/

The Health News and Information Directory

Comprehensive resource indexed by medical condition. Gives current news on the condition or illness and provides links to further information.
World Wide Web URL: http://www.healthnewsdirectory.com/HealthNews/ Directory/Default.asp?Reference=HealthNews.Categories%3A0

Health care HeadlineNews

HeadlineNews is a comprehensive, Web-based health care news service. Health care headlines are categorized into over 150 news topics. Links to the full news stories are provided on each page.
World Wide Web URL: http://www.achoo.com/news/default.asp

Healthline—USA Today Health Stories

Daily news feed of *USA Today* stories.
World Wide Web URL: http://usatoday.com/life/health/lhd1.htm

Internet FDA

An electronic source of information about the U.S. Food and Drug Administration.
World Wide Web URL: http://www.fda.gov/

Los Alamos National Laboratory Home Page

Los Alamos National Laboratory has a diverse set of research projects ongoing at any one time. For the doctor or medical researcher, the projects of interest may range from telemedicine or genetics databases to flow cytometry. Search or browse through over 100 servers with tens of thousands of documents.
World Wide Web URL: http://www.lanl.gov/worldview/

Medical Breakthroughs Reported by Ivanhoe Broadcast News

This content-driven, multimedia site highlights three reports per week on breakthroughs from the world· of medicine. Presented by Ivanhoe Broadcast News, the site offers a keyword search of subjects, rotating topics like Woman

To Woman and Dr.'s Q&A, a free e-mail bulletin listing topics to come, and an archive of medical news in categories.
World Wide Web URL: http://www.ivanhoe.com

Reuters Health Information Services and Medical News

Professionally targeted medical news provided for a subscription fee. Updated daily and full-text searchable. The site includes articles grouped under the following headings: clinical, economic, epidemiology, legislative, legal, policy, professional development, regulatory, and science. Requires paid subscription.
World Wide Web URL: http://www.reutershealth.com

The Universe of Women's Health

A physician-reviewed service offering medical professionals, women, and industry a home for publishing, accessing information, and global interaction. It offers three sections, each focusing on different segments of the women's health community: medical professionals, medical industry, and women.
World Wide Web URL: http://www.obgyn.net/medical.asp

Your Health Daily from the New York Times

Archive of articles that cover news and developments on AIDS, Alzheimer's, arthritis, asthma, etc. Designed for a general audience or patient education. Includes articles culled from the "Your Health Daily" archives organized by disease. From AIDS to women's health, also includes topic headings for men's health, childcare, cholesterol, dental health, elderly, nutrition/exercises, sexual health, stroke, and more.
World Wide Web URL: http://yourhealthdaily.com/

Associations and Societies

American Academy of Dermatology

This is the home page for the American Academy of Dermatology. It offers patient and professional information, including a physician finding service and continuing education opportunities for its members.
World Wide Web URL: http://www.aad.org

American Academy of Family Physicians

Like most organizational sites, this one provides members and public resources in its areas of interest. Continuing medical education, publications, news, and up-coming meeting information is also provided.
World Wide Web URL: http://www.aafp.org/

American Academy of Neurology

The American Academy of Neurology home page.
World Wide Web URL: http://www.aan.com/

American Academy of Orthopaedic Surgeons

This site provides both member and public access to topics of interest to orthopedists and patients with orthopedic concerns. Included are directories of specialists, an orthopedic yellow pages, and information about meetings. Links to other medical sites and Medline are available.
World Wide Web URL: http://www.aaos.org

American Academy of Otolaryngology—Head and Neck Surgery

The AAO-HNS site provides patient indicators, a virtual museum, research pages, and access to its journal, *Otolaryngology—Head and Neck Surgery*. The virtual museum includes such topics as hearing aids through the ages and the role of African Americans in the specialty.
World Wide Web URL: http://www.entnet.org/

American Academy of Pediatrics

Topics and membership benefits for the members of the American Academy of Pediatrics.
World Wide Web URL: http://www.aap.org

American Association of Clinical Endocrinologists

The American Association of Clinical Endocrinologists is a professional medical organization devoted to the field of clinical endocrinology. Its mission is to enhance the practice of clinical endocrinology.
World Wide Web URL: http://www.aace.com/

American Association of Health Plans

This site is provided by a trade organization representing HMOs.
World Wide Web URL: http://www.aahp.org

American Association of Respiratory Care

Home page for the American Association of Respiratory Care. It contains information and resources for health care professionals and AARC members.
World Wide Web URL: http://www.AARC.org

American Board of Internal Medicine

The American Board of Internal Medicine Web site offers information about the board, its functions as a certifying body, and upcoming certifying examinations.
World Wide Web URL: http://www.abim.org

American Cancer Society

This site offers local and national cancer news and the ability to search the site for specific content. It includes a media services section that is interesting and a useful source of information for those in the media.
World Wide Web URL: http://www.cancer.org

American College of Cardiology

Designed mainly for members, this site provides news and updates, continuing education, self-assessment programs, and meeting information.
World Wide Web URL: http://www.acc.org

American College of Emergency Physicians

Member services and information for members of the American College of Emergency Physicians.
World Wide Web URL: http://www.cep.org/

American College of Nurse-Midwives

Contains information about nurse-midwifery practice, how to find nurse-midwives, ACNM chapters, nurse-midwifery education programs, and the ACNM news journal, *Quickening*.
World Wide Web URL: http://www.acnm.org/

American College of Physicians (ACP)

American College of Physicians (ACP) provides selections from ACP journals; CME, medical computing, managed care information; classifieds; Web site reviews; product catalog; and more.
World Wide Web URL: http://www.acponline.org/

American College of Physician Executives

Founded in 1975 as the American Academy of Medical Directors, the American College of Physician Executives has grown to more than 12,000 physician members—a unique group of physicians who directly influence the path of health care in America. The college's members are physician executives with management or administrative responsibilities in hospitals, group practices, managed care, government, universities, the military, and industry. The site includes information for members and nonmembers with an interest in these areas.
World Wide Web URL: http://www.acpe.org

The American College of Obstetricians and Gynecolgists

Offers searchable access to publications and educational materials. Requires registration (free), though some public access is permitted.
World Wide Web URL: http://www.acog.org/

American Gastroenterological Association

Home page for the American Gastroenterological Association.
World Wide Web URL: http://www.gastro.org/

American Health Decisions

American Health Decisions is a confederation of state health programs that assists in developing education programs about health care and policy. The group promotes patients' rights in medical care, including the right to refuse or accept treatment. It also conducts research on health care policy issues.
World Wide Web URL: http://www.ahd.org

American Lung Association

A searchable site with information about smoking, radon, and various lung diseases.
World Wide Web URL: http://www.lungusa.org/

American Medical Association

Web site of the American Medical Association. Provides health and fitness info for resources on conditions and family health.
World Wide Web URL: http://www.ama-assn.org

American Medical Informatics Association

This Web site is designed to help answer questions about AMIA, its services, and activities. At this Web site, you can find out about meetings and educational events, membership in AMIA, AMIA's structure and operations, publications, medical informatics and related issues, and background information about previous meetings.
World Wide Web URL: http://amia2.amia.org/

American Medical Women's Association

This national organization supports the advancement of women in medicine and the improvement of women's health. The site lists women's health books, publications, and provides information about various health topics.
World Wide Web URL: http://www.amwa-doc.org

American Physical Therapy Association

This site offers information for patients and physical therapists alike. Links to other Internet resources and the Amazon Books site provide additional information.
World Wide Web URL: http://www.apta.org

American Psychological Association

This is the Internet service of the American Psychological Association. It has a great deal of material here for the public and APA members. "What You Should Know About Women and Depression" is just one of the valuable articles available at the APA site.
World Wide Web URL: http://www.apa.org/

American Society for Reproductive Medicine

Formerly the American Fertility Society, this nonprofit scientific organization addresses all aspects of female and male reproduction, and endorses NAMS consumer education materials.
World Wide Web URL: http://www.asrm.com

American Telemedicine Association

Established in 1993 as a nonprofit organization and headquartered in Washington, DC, membership in the association is open to individuals, companies, and other organizations with an interest in promoting the deployment of telemedicine throughout the United States and worldwide. The site offers a members-only side and a public side, including a yet to be implemented section on e-health.

World Wide Web URL: http://www.atmeda.org/

American Urological Association

A member site that contains advanced graphics such as java and animated GIFs. Public and members-only information is available, along with an on-line museum.

World Wide Web URL: http://www.auanet.org/

American Urological Society

Dedicated to improving the care for women with lower urinary tract disorders, the society offers help locating a practitioner, as well as general information about incontinence.

World Wide Web URL: http://www.augs.org/

The Arthritis Foundation

Extensive information for patients and parents of patients with arthritis. The site contains a large number of links to relevant information and other sites.

World Wide Web URL: http://www.arthritis.org/

Association of Professors of Obstetrics and Gynecology

This site offers members information about meetings, publications, and academic positions that are available. This site was a good example of the need to type the ".org" on the end of the URL or you could end up somewhere you didn't expect—apgo.com at one time led to a pornography site.

World Wide Web URL: http://www.apgo.org

Brookings Institution

Brookings Institution is a nonprofit research organization that examines current and emerging policy challenges and offers recommendations for dealing with them. It supports extensive research programs. Brookings seeks to improve the performance of American institutions, the effectiveness of government programs, and the quality of U.S. public policies. It addresses current and emerging policy challenges and offers practical recommendations for dealing with them, expressed in language that is accessible to policymakers and the general public alike.

World Wide Web URL: http://www.brook.edu

Canadian Cancer Society

The leading Canadian nonprofit organization focusing on education about cancer prevention and treatment.

World Wide Web URL: http://www.cancer.ca

Eyenet

This site is the official site for the American Academy of Ophthalmology. This searchable site even includes the option to send and receive e-mail from the site of their annual meeting.

World Wide Web URL: http://www.eyenet.org/

The Juvenile Diabetes Foundation

The Juvenile Diabetes Foundation is a not-for-profit, voluntary health agency whose mission is to support and fund research to find a cure for diabetes and its complications.

World Wide Web URL: http://www.jdrf.org/

Medic Alert

Information about the MedicAlert system.

World Wide Web URL: http://www.medicalert.org/

National Association of Public Hospitals and Health Systems

The National Association of Public Hospitals and Health Systems is an organization that represents the nation's urban public hospitals, health systems, and the people they serve. Its mission is to educate the public and policymakers about the challenges facing public hospitals and the populations they serve. It is an advocate for health care reform that would improve insurance coverage, access to health care, and the general well-being of those who are the most vulnerable participants in the nation's health system.

World Wide Web URL: http://www.naph.org

National Association of Social Workers

A nonprofit organization for U.S. health care professionals in this specialty.
World Wide Web URL: http://www.naswdc.org

National Board of Respiratory Care

The home page for the voluntary health certifying board that was created in 1960 to evaluate the professional competence of respiratory therapists.
World Wide Web URL: http://www.nbrc.org/

National Institute on Aging (NIA)

The NIA offers brochures and fact sheets regarding health and aging, including diseases/conditions, health promotion and disease prevention, medical care, medications and immunizations, nutrition, and safety.
World Wide Web URL: http://www.nih.gov/nia/

National Mental Health Association

Facts, figures, and discussions about mental illness in the family, depression, schizophrenia, anxiety disorders, and more are provided here by the NMHA.
World Wide Web URL: http://www.nmha.org

North American Menopause Society

The NAMS Web site deals with issues about menopause, including information about the society. It contains information, publications, and links related to menopause.
World Wide Web URL: http://www.menopause.org/

Nursing World

Nursing World is sponsored by the American Nurses Association and offers links to products, services, journals, continuing education, and more.
World Wide Web URL: http://www.nursingworld.org

Osteoporosis and Related Bone Diseases National Resource Center

This site is your complete source for osteoporosis information including details about Paget's disease of bone and osteogenesis imperfecta. It's supported by the National Institute of Arthritis and Musculoskeletal and Skin Diseases.
World Wide Web URL: http://www.osteo.org/

Planned Parenthood

Looking for resources on sexual and reproductive health, family planning, STDs, or sexuality education? The home page for Planned Parenthood includes education resources for a variety of audiences on these topics, and more, as well as extensive links to related organizations. The site offers a Spanish-language option as well.
World Wide Web URL: http://www.plannedparenthood.org/

Plastic Surgery Information Center

The Web site for plastic surgery is sponsored by the American Society of Plastic and Reconstructive Surgeons (ASPRS) and the Plastic Surgery Educational Foundation (PSEF). This site provides background on the wide variety of cosmetic and reconstructive plastic surgery procedures as well as offering a plastic surgeon referral service. There is also information on ASPRS, PSEF, and other plastic surgery organizations.
World Wide Web URL: http://www.plasticsurgery.org/

Royal College of Physicians and Surgeons of Canada

The Royal College of Physicians and Surgeons of Canada offers this site in both English and French for its members.
World Wide Web URL: http://rcpsc.medical.org/

Royal Society of Medicine

The Internet is truly international. This is the site of the Royal Society of Medicine in the United Kingdom. Like other association home pages, this site provides services to its members, access to publications, and limited information for the public.
World Wide Web URL: http://www.roysocmed.ac.uk/

Society for Endocrinology

The Society for Endocrinology aims to promote the advancement of public education in endocrinology.
World Wide Web URL: http://www.endocrinology.org/

Society of Obstetricians and Gynaecologists of Canada

The Society of Obstetricians and Gynaecologists of Canada provides information and services for its members and the public through this site.
World Wide Web URL: http://www.sogc.org/SOGCnet/index_e.shtml

Society for Reproductive Endocrinology and Infertility

This site offers a geographic index to members and a link to the American Society of Reproductive Medicine.
World Wide Web URL: http://www.socrei.org/

Society of General Internal Medicine

The Society of General Internal Medicine was founded to promote improved patient care, research, and education in primary care. The Web site provides information about the group and links to other sites of possible interest.
World Wide Web URL: http://www.sgim.org/

Society of Gynecologic Oncologists

Here you will find an introduction to the specialty of gynecologic oncology and information about gynecological cancers from the SGO.
World Wide Web URL: http://www.sgo.org/

The Society of Throacic Surgeons

With both member and public sides, this site offers video clips and a link to an on-line full-text and graphics version of the *Annals of Throacic Surgery*.
World Wide Web URL: http://www.sts.org/

World Health Organization

The home page of the World Wide Web InfoServer of WHO, among the UN systems and the major international organizations in Geneva, Switzerland. For comprehensive background information on world health data, this site is invaluable. Includes a Weekly Epidemiological Record with access to back copies and a Statistical Information System that covers a range of diseases as well as public health categories of risk.
World Wide Web URL: http://www.who.org/

History and Reference

Health Care Financing Administration

The Health Care Financing Administration is the federal agency that oversees Medicare and Medicaid. This site provides information about programs, rules, regulations, and research associated with its mission.
World Wide Web URL: http://www.hcfa.gov

Inner Learning Guide

The Inner Learning Guide is the place for fun, interactive, and educational views of the human body. This program contains over 100 illustrations of the human body with animations and thousands of descriptive links. Human Anatomy On-line uses Java applets to show images and selected anatomy parts.
World Wide Web URL: http://www.innerbody.com/htm/body.html

Merck Manual (17th edition)

The 17th edition of the famous *Merck Manual* is the centennial edition. It is available on-line and the site provides search capabilities to make its use easier.
World Wide Web URL: http://www.merck.com/pubs/mmanual/

Multilingual Glossary of Technical and Popular Medical Terms in Nine European Languages

List consists of 1,830 terms that are translated into seven other languages. Terms and glossary may be browsed by language. This project was commissioned by the European Commission (DG III) and executed by Heymans Institute of Pharmacology and Mercator School, Department of Applied Linguistics.
World Wide Web URL: http://allserv.rug.ac.be/~rvdstich/eugloss/welcome.html

Museum of Questionable Medical Devices

Bob McCoy, the site operator, is a veritable encyclopedia of the world's most inane and useless information about how to cure and/or comprehend what may ail or puzzle you. He is shown getting aphrenology reading (the machine measures the size of bumps on the head). The reading lets him know how he's doing on any of 35 personality characteristics like intelligence, spirituality, suavity, and chastity. The site includes pictures of electric shock machines and a foot-powered breast enlarger. These are only a sample of the many devices and practices that are illustrated at this interesting site.
World Wide Web URL: http://www.mtn.org/~quack/

U.S. National Library of Medicine

Entry point for the National Library of Medicine including general information, databases, and photographic archives. Connections to comprehensive databases of medical information such as MEDLARS and MEDLINE are also available.
World Wide Web URL: http://www.nlm.nih.gov/

The Visible Embryo

Welcome to the Visible Embryo, a comprehensive resource of information on human development from conception to birth, designed for both medical student and interested lay people. The Visible Embryo offers a detailed pictorial account of normal and abnormal development. The Visible Embryo teaches the first 4 weeks of human development from fertilization to somite development. Great graphics and movies are offered.
World Wide Web URL: http://visembryo.com

The Visible Human Project

The Visible Human Project is an outgrowth of the NLM's 1986 long-range plan. It is creating a complete, anatomically detailed, three-dimensional representations of the male and female human body. The current phase of the project is collecting transverse CT, MRI, and cryosection images of representative male and female cadavers at 1-mm intervals. This site offers information and images from this project.
World Wide Web URL: http://www.nlm.nih.gov/research/visible/ visible_human.html

The Whole Brain Atlas

An impressive site that contains thousands of images of the normal brain and 32 medical conditions, from Alzheimer's disease to stroke and multiple sclerosis. The site allows one to zoom through brain slices, see movies that follow a patient's condition over time, and superimpose images made using different modalities.
World Wide Web URL: http://www.med.harvard.edu/AANLIB/home.html

Computers and Health

Department of Medical Informatics

Here you can find the most relevant links to Web sites on health informatics. Simply choose a country from the index and the links to that particular country will appear.
World Wide Web URL: http://www.imbi.uni-freiburg.de/medinf/ mi_list.htm

Ancillary Support

Multilingual Glossary of Medical Terms

This project was commissioned by the European Commission (DG III) and executed by Heymans Institute of Pharmacology and Mercator School, Department of Applied Linguistics. It covers nine languages!
World Wide Web URL: http://allserv.rug.ac.be/~rvdstich/eugloss/ welcome.html

Practice and Patients

Patient Education

Family Doctor

This site is provided by the American Academy of Family Practice and contains health information in both categorized and searchable formats.
World Wide Web URL: http://www.familydoctor.org

I Am Growing

This commercial site started by a pair of obstetricians offers a personalized calendar with information about a patient's growing pregnancy.
World Wide Web URL: http://www.iamgrowing.com

MDChoice.com

The former NetMedicine.com site, this site offers portals for both patients and physicians.
World Wide Web URL: http://www.mdchoice.com

Medifor Inc.

This Internet service offers customizable patient education materials to supplement physicians' care instructions in over 800 primary care topics. It offers links to related sites.
World Wide Web URL: http://www.medifor.com

Medinotes

This site provides information and contact points for the Charting Plus 4 electronic medical record system offered by Medinotes.
World Wide Web URL: http://www.medinotes.com/home.htm

The Patient Education Institute

The Patient Education Institute offers software and hardware services to health care institutions interested in implementing interactive health communication systems for patient education, informed consent, health promotion, patient satisfaction survey, patient medical history, and service promotion.
World Wide Web URL: http://www.patient-education.com

The Virtual Hospital

Virtual Hospital is a service of University of Iowa Health Care, providing patient and physician information and links.
World Wide Web URL: http://www.vh.org

Practice Management or Marketing

Mednetrix.com

This company offers to help develop a Web site for you that is customized to an individual medical practice and its medical specialty. You control the content.
World Wide Web URL: http://www.mednetrix.com

Medscape

Medscape offers an electronic record system that includes digital health records, and allows access anytime and anywhere a physician-patient encounter takes place. As of June 2000, more than 13 million patient records had been created with this system. This site gives overviews of the system and a demonstration.
World Wide Web URL: http://www.medicalogic.com

Medical Reference and Disease Specific Sites

Medical Internet Guides

Medscape Today

A general medical Internet site with links to news, CME offerings, and disease specific information. The site offers customized information for medical students, officer managers, nurses, and others. Registration is required.
World Wide Web URL: http://www.medscape.com

General

The Argus Clearinghouse

The Health and Medicine category includes guides on topics pertaining to the general condition and well-being of body and mind, and to the study and practice of maintaining and improving health, as well as the prevention or treatment of diseases and disorders.
World Wide Web URL: http://www.clearinghouse.net/cgi-bin/chadmin/ viewcat/Health___Medicine?kywd++

Ask NOAH

This is a general health information site. New York Online Access to Health (NOAH) is a project that brought together the unique assets and experience of four New York partners who have worked together on a variety of projects for 26 years: the City University of New York, the Metropolitan New York Library Council, the New York Academy of Medicine, and the New York Public Library. The information provided is available in both English and Spanish.
World Wide Web URL: http://www.noah-health.org/

Drug InforNet

This private Health On the Net Foundation subscriber, offers a wide variety of drug-related information for both providers and patients alike. The site contains searchable databases of information taken from both the professional and patient package inserts. The information is available by brand name, generic name, manufacturer, and therapeutic class. Beyond the drug-related information supplied are links to other sites for information about diseases, medical news items, medical schools, government agencies, and hospitals.
World Wide Web URL: http://www.druginfonet.com

Health Resources and Services Administration

The Health Resources and Services Administration has compiled a directory of health-related information for cities around the United States. The site is easy to move around, making comparisons easy to do for data from various cities or regions.
World Wide Web URL: http://www.hrsa.gov

National Center for Biotechnology Information

Established in 1988 as a national resource for molecular biology information, NCBI creates public databases, conducts research in computational biology, develops software tools for analyzing genome data, and disseminates biomedical information—all for the better understanding of molecular processes affecting human health and disease. This is its entry point for Internet information.
World Wide Web URL: http://www.ncbi.nlm.nih.gov

Virtual Human

Still under development, the Virtual Human Gallery will be re-released in Spring 2001 as one of the world's premier collections of scientifically accurate 3D anatomical imagery, animations, and multimedia. The involved medical illustration and programming teams are rapidly building the new site, which will offer the opportunity to browse and link to (for free) or download (for a fee) a comprehensive collection of content for education, teaching, presentation, and other needs.
World Wide Web URL: http://vhgallery.gsm.com/

The Wellcome Trust

The Wellcome Trust a wide-ranging collection of health-related information on a variety of topics. The site offers current information and special "exhibits" as well as a searchable database.
World Wide Web URL: http://www.wellcome.ac.uk

Cases

MDChoice Cyberpatient simulator

A pair of offerings supplied by the MDChoice, these simulators give you a chance to try your skill at cardiac resuscitation.
World Wide Web URL: http://www.mdchoice.com/cyberpt/cyber.asp

Addiction and Substance Abuse

Al-Anon/Alateen

The goal of Al-Anon/Alateen is to help families and friends of alcoholics recover from the effects of living with the problem drinking of a relative or friend. Alateen, is the recovery program for young people. Alateen groups are sponsored by Al-Anon members. Information and connections to local groups are available at this site.
World Wide Web URL: http://www.al-anon-alateen.org/

Alcoholics Anonymous

The site provides general and contact information for Alcoholics Anonymous and 12-step program services in the United States, Canada, and other locations. The site is available in English, Spanish, and French.
World Wide Web URL: http://www.alcoholics-anonymous.org

Cocaine Anonymous World Services

The Escape Cocaine site promotes the 12-Step Recovery Program and provides information about cocaine, crack, and other mind-altering substances.
World Wide Web URL: http://www.ca.org

Minnesota Higher Education Center Against Violence and Abuse

This violence and abuse clearinghouse includes education and training resources, bibliographies, papers, reports, art, poetry, and a comprehensive list of related Web links.
World Wide Web URL: http://www.mincava.umn.edu

National Clearinghouse for Alcohol and Drug Information (NCADI)

NCADI provides on-line forums, referrals, searchable databases, research, statistics, publications, resources, and links relevant to substance abuse and mental health sites.
World Wide Web URL: http://www.health.org

National Council on Alcoholism and Drug Dependence, Inc.

Parents and children will find information about alcoholism and drug addictions, resources, and referrals at the NCADD's site. The council advocates the prevention, intervention, research, and treatment of alcoholism and drug dependence.
World Wide Web URL: http://www.ncadd.org

National Institute on Alcohol Abuse and Alcoholism

Publications, resources, and databases pertaining to alcoholism and alcohol abuse are available through the NIAAA.
World Wide Web URL: http://www.niaaa.nih.gov/

National Institute on Drug Abuse

NIDA provides information about drugs of abuse, offers search capabilities, provides publications, and includes links to other related sites.
World Wide Web URL: http://www.nida.nih.gov

Violence Against Women Office

Information about domestic violence, related federal legislation, ongoing research and studies, and selected articles is provided by the Violence Against Women Office, as well as a link to the National Domestic Violence Hotline.
World Wide Web URL: http://www.ojp.usdoj.gov/vawo/

Aging and Gerontology

American Association of Retired Persons

"AARP, celebrating 40 years of service to Americans of all ages, is the nation's leading organization for people age 50 and older. It serves their needs and interests through information and education advocacy, and community services that are provided by a network of local chapters and experienced volunteers through-

out the country." The organization also offers members a wide range of special benefits and services, including *Modern Maturity* magazine and the monthly *Bulletin*.
World Wide Web URL: http://www.aarp.org/

Geriatrics

Access to the journal *Geriatrics* is available at this site.
World Wide Web URL: http://www.geri.com/

National Institute on Aging (NIA)

The NIA offers brochures and fact sheets regarding health and aging, including diseases/conditions, health promotion and disease prevention, medical care, medications and immunizations, nutrition and safety.
World Wide Web URL: http://www.nih.gov/nia/

North American Menopause Society

The NAMS Web site deals with issues about menopause, including information about the society. It contains information, publications, and links related to menopause.
World Wide Web URL: http://www.menopause.org/

AIDS

Aaron Diamond AIDS Research Center

This is the site for the Aaron Diamond AIDS Research Center of New York and the site is supported by a grant from Galaxo Wellcome Pharmaceuticals.
World Wide Web URL: http://www.adarc.org/

Ægis

This patient-oriented site is considered the largest AIDS/HIV database in the world. Includes top related news story for the day, and advice if you think you are at risk.
World Wide Web URL: http://www.aegis.com/

AIDS

This site is listed as "Shared Rights, Shared Responsibilities" and is a loose collection of information about AIDS and lifestyles. An interesting jumping-off point for patients and medical personnel alike.
World Wide Web URL: http://www.iohk.com/UserPages/mlau/
aidshome.html

AIDS Resource List

AIDS Resource List has many links to all kinds of HIV/AIDS-related sites.
World Wide Web URL: http://www.specialweb.com/aids/

AIDS Virtual Library

A frequently updated library of information and links to information about HIV and AIDS. This virtual library deals with the social, political, and medical aspects of AIDS, HIV, and related issues. This site is maintained on a volunteer basis, so updates are subject to availability.
World Wide Web URL: http://Quniverse.com/aidsvl/

CDC National AIDS Clearinghouse

The CDC National AIDS Clearinghouse's services are designed to facilitate the sharing of HIV/AIDS and STD resources and information about education and prevention, published materials, and research findings, as well as news about related trends. The CDC National AIDS Clearinghouse is a service of the Centers for Disease Control and Prevention.
World Wide Web URL: http://www.maghrebnet.net.ma/alcs/links/
cdcnac_aspensys_com.html

The Center for AIDS Prevention Studies (CAPS)

The Center for AIDS Prevention Studies (CAPS) conducts epidemiological and behavioral studies in the primary prevention and early intervention of HIV disease. Here you'll find fact sheets, descriptions of effective prevention pro-

grams, CAPS faculty and staff, CAPS prevention publications, news releases, job and research opportunities at CAPS, and more.
World Wide Web URL: http://www.caps.ucsf.edu/

Guide to NIH HIV/AIDS Information Services

In this guide, the National Library of Medicine draws together in a single, easy-to-use source, a variety of data about the many HIV/AIDS information-related activities of NIH along with selected PHS offerings. The guide was first prepared for the NIH HIV/AIDS Information Services Conference, co-sponsored by the National Library of Medicine and the NIH Office of AIDS Research, in June 1993.

World Wide Web URL: http://sis.nlm.nih.gov/aids/index.html

HIV Information Network

This site offers a number of continuing education and information options including a fax newsletter, ask the experts, news, meetings, discussion groups, and clinical rounds. A number of links to other HIV sites is also provided.

World Wide Web URL: http://www.hivline.com

HIV Insite

Hosted by the University of California, San Francisco, this site bills itself as a "gateway to AIDS knowledge." The site aims to improve on government AIDS sites both in look and content. The site has links to a huge range of material from news on drug studies to audio reports from recent conferences. The site also includes the AIDS Knowledge Base.

World Wide Web URL: http://hivinsite.ucsf.edu/

HIV.net

Information on HIV and AIDS that is continuously updated. This site is also available in German.

World Wide Web URL: http://hiv.net

JAMA HIV/AIDS Information Center

Detailed information about HIV and AIDS including news articles and Web links, this site provides an easy-to-use, interactive collection of useful and high-quality resources for physicians, other health professionals, and the public. The links will let you access clinical updates, news, and information on a broad range of social and policy questions relating to HIV/AIDS. This site is made possible by an unrestricted educational grant from GlaxoWellcome. It is produced by staff of the *Journal of the American Medical Association* under the direction of an editorial review panel of leading HIV/AIDS authorities.

World Wide Web URL: http://www.ama-assn.org/special/hiv/hivhome.htm

National Library of Medicine AIDS Resources

A set of links to resources about HIV and AIDS.
World Wide Web URL: http://sis.nlm.nih.gov/hiv.cfm

Positive Action

Funded in partnership with Glaxo Wellcome, Positive Action was started to provide community education and support for HIV and AIDS. The Positive Action site is designed to provide ongoing access to information about Positive Action activities, to encourage participation and comment through its feedback site and discussion forum, and to assist in formulating new ideas for future projects and areas of collaboration.
World Wide Web URL: http://www.positiveaction.com/

Positive.org

Positive.org is dedicated to having a positive attitude about sexuality—gay, straight, or bi. It stresses safe sexuality and reinforces the idea that there's nothing wrong with you if you decide to have sex, and nothing wrong with you if you decide not to. The site has many topics, a glossary, and search capabilities. Site maintained by the Coalition for Positive Sexuality. (A Spanish-language version is also available.)
World Wide Web URL: http://www.positive.org/Home/index.html

The Safer Sex Page

This is the largest archive of information on safe sex information on the World Wide Web.
World Wide Web URL: http://www.safersex.org/

The Terrence Higgins Trust

The Terrence Higgins Trust is a national, London-based, nongovernmental organization. It was set up in 1982 to provide information and support to people living with HIV and AIDS, and to people affected or concerned. The site offers a variety of support and information resources.
World Wide Web URL: http://www.tht.org.uk/

Allergy

Allergy and Asthma Rochester Resource Center (AARRC)

The mission of the Allergy and Asthma Rochester Resource Center is to improve the health of children and adults who suffer from allergies and asthma by providing didactic and practical learning experiences for physicians in training, primary care physicians, nurses, pharmacists, and other health care professionals; by providing learning and service activities for adults and children with allergies and asthma to help them to cope with and to self-manage their allergic and asthmatic conditions; and by conducting clinical research using a large patient base with the full spectrum of allergic and asthmatic conditions.
World Wide Web URL: http://www.aarrc.com

Allergy Asthma Technology, Inc.

Allergy Asthma Technology is committed to providing the most up-to-date, medically approved products available, and have established relationships with various health care organizations that provide health information that can be passed on to consumers. (Commercial site)
World Wide Web URL: http://allergyasthmatech.com

American Academy of Allergy Asthma and Immunology

Representing allergists, clinical immunologists, and allied health professionals, the AAAAI provides general information, physician referrals, and answers to frequently asked questions. The site offers information about topics of interest, up-coming meetings, and the ability to submit abstracts on-line. Its Web page contains information for patients and physicians, though its content is directed mainly at professionals. If you're wondering how asthma affects pregnancy or what are the best pets for a person with allergies, this is the site to hit.
World Wide Web URL: http://www.aaaai.org

American College of Allergy, Asthma, and Immunology On-line

The American College of Allergy, Asthma, and Immunology is a professional organization representing the scientific and other interests of allergist-immunologists. Its Web page contains information for patients and physicians.
World Wide Web URL: http://allergy.mcg.edu/

Food Allergy Network

The Food Allergy Network (FAN) is a nonprofit organization established to help families living with food allergies, and to increase public awareness about food

allergies and anaphylaxis. FAN provides education, emotional support, and coping strategies.
World Wide Web URL: http://www.foodallergy.org/

National Institute of Allergy and Infectious Diseases

This site offers searchable information about the National Institute of Allergy and Infectious Diseases, educational and research programs offered, and links to other related sites.
World Wide Web URL: http://www.niaid.nih.gov/

Alternative Medicine

Acupuncture.com/

This site offers information about the traditional oriental therapies of acupuncture, herbology, Qi Gong, Chinese nutrition, Tui Na and Chinese massage, and Chinese diagnostic methods. Information is provided for consumers, practitioners, and students.
World Wide Web URL: http://www.Acupuncture.com/

Alternative Medicine Home Page

The Alternative Medicine Home Page is a jump station for sources of information on unconventional, unorthodox, unproven or alternative, complementary, innovative, integrative therapies. When visited around the first of the year, the site had not been updated since August, but still contained a group of useful and current links.
World Wide Web URL: http://www.pitt.edu/~cbw/altm.html

Aesclepian Chronicles

A collection of papers and information about the Synergistic Health Center in Chapel Hill, North Carolina.
World Wide Web URL: http://www.forthrt.com/~chronicl

Ask Dr. Weil

Dr. Andrew Weil, author of *Spontaneous Healing*, is an advocate of integrating Western medicine with homeopathy and other alternative treatments. His site (which launched on HotWired in 1996 and moved to Time's Pathfinder in 1997) offers a daily Q&A, a database of symptoms and conditions, an 8-week health program, and a vitamin adviser.
World Wide Web URL: http://drweil.com/

Bradley Method of Natural Childbirth

Information about the Bradley method of natural childbirth and husband-coached childbirth.
World Wide Web URL: http://www.bradleybirth.com/

Chiropractic OnLine

Chiropractic OnLine is presented as a public service by the American Chiropractic Association and contains a long list of resources for consumers, health professionals, and others.
World Wide Web URL: http://www.amerchiro.org/

Good Medicine Magazine

A source for alternative medicine information and exchange.
World Wide Web URL: http://coolware.com/health/medical_reporter/ health.html

Homeopathy Home Page

This page is a central jumping-off point and aims to provide links to related resources. Graphics are kept to a minimum on this site.
World Wide Web URL: http://www.homeopathyhome.com

NIH Office of Alternative Medicine

The National Institutes of Health offers information on alternative and complementary medicines, and details of research results.
World Wide Web URL: http://nccam.nih.gov/

Scientific Research on the Transcendental Meditation Program

A compilation of over 500 studies that have been completed on the physiological, psychological, and sociological effects of Maharishi's transcendental meditation and TM-Sidhi programs.
World Wide Web URL: http://www.mum.edu/tm_program/welcome.html

Alzheimer's Disease

Alzheimer's association

The Alzheimer's Association site provides links to local chapters, information for families and providers, and information about research opportunities, grants, and deadlines.
World Wide Web URL: http://www.alz.org/

ALZHEIMER Page

The ALZHEIMER Page is an educational service created and sponsored by the Washington University Alzheimer's Disease Research Center (ADRC) in St. Louis, Missouri and supported by a grant from the National Institute on Aging.
World Wide Web URL: http://www.biostat.wustl.edu/ALZHEIMER

Alzheimer's Disease Education and Referral Center

The Alzheimer's Disease Education and Referral (ADEAR) Center's Web site contains information, referral, and publications. The ADEAR Center is a service of the National Institute on Aging (NIA). The NIA is one of the National Institutes of Health, under the U.S. Department of Health and Human Services.
World Wide Web URL: http://www.alzheimers.org/

The Whole Brain Atlas

An impressive site that contains thousands of images of the normal brain and 32 medical conditions, from Alzheimer's disease to stroke and multiple sclerosis. The site allows one to zoom through brain slices, see movies that follow a patient's condition over time, and superimpose images made using different modalities.
World Wide Web URL: http://www.med.harvard.edu/AANLIB/home.html

Assault (Physical and Sexual Abuse)

Rape, Abuse and Incest National Network

A clearinghouse for information about and for victims of rape, abuse, and incest.
World Wide Web URL: http://rainn.org/

Sexual Assault Information Page

A searchable list of resources and sites.
World Wide Web URL: http://www.cs.utk.edu/~bartley/saInfoPage.html

Asthma

American Academy of Allergy, Asthma & Immunology

The American Academy of Allergy, Asthma & Immunology site offers information about topics of interest, up-coming meetings, and the ability to submit abstracts on-line. Its Web page contains information for patients and physicians, though its content is directed mainly at professionals.
World Wide Web URL: http://www.aaaai.org

American College of Allergy, Asthma & Immunology On-line

The American College of Allergy, Asthma & Immunology is a professional organization representing the scientific and other interests of allergist-immunologists. Its Web page contains information for patients and physicians.
World Wide Web URL: http://allergy.mcg.edu/

Dundee University Asthma Research Unit Home Page

The aim of the Asthma Research Unit is to produce high-quality research in the treatment and management of patients with asthma. "Until such a time as the laboratories produce a 'cure' for asthma, we believe it is work such as ours that can best benefit the patient. By educating medical staff through dissemination of our findings we can help ensure that all patients with asthma receive the best possible care."
World Wide Web URL: http://www.dundee.ac.uk/GeneralPractice/Asthma/

Global Initiative for Asthma

A collaboration between the National Heart, Lung, and Blood Institute, the World Health Organization, and the National Institutes on Health. Provides multiformat full-text versions of the 1993 Workshop Report: Global Strategy for Asthma Management and Prevention, as well as guides to asthma management and a patient guide.
World Wide Web URL: http://www.ginasthma.com/

Breast Disease

Breast Cancer Information Clearinghouse

A repository for current information about breast cancer funded by the New York State Science and Technology Foundation (NYSERNet). NYSERNet, Inc. established the Breast Cancer Information Clearinghouse in 1994 at a time when there was little or no useful content on the Internet for a breast cancer patient. The BCIC was formed as a partnership of local and national organizations dedicated to the fight of this disease. These organizations provided the content for the site, and NYSERNet provided the tools and technology necessary to make this information available to the world.
World Wide Web URL: http://www.nabco.org/resources/

Breast Cancer Roundtable

This site is devoted to issues concerning breast cancer, and contains information from many on-line journals, research studies, and organizations. A new issue will be presented each month. Your opinion may be inputted.
World Wide Web URL: http://www.seas.gwu.edu/student/tlooms/ MGT243/bcr.html

Breast Diseases—Multimedia Course Work—McGill

A comprehensive site dealing with breast disease from anatomy to clinical management. Designed for third-year medical students and presented by McGill University.
World Wide Web URL: http://mystic.biomed.mcgill.ca/MedinfHome/ MedInf/Breastcourse/htmltext/home/BreastHome.html

Community Breast Health Project (CBHP)

The mission of the Community Breast Health Project is to improve the lives of people touched by breast cancer by acting as a clearinghouse for information and support, providing volunteer opportunities for breast cancer survivors and friends dedicated to helping others with the disease, and serving as an educational resource and a community center for all who are concerned about breast cancer and breast health. The Community Breast Health Project is grass-roots, patient-driven, and committed to providing services free of charge.
World Wide Web URL: http://www-med.stanford.edu/CBHP/

Cornell University Program on Breast Cancer and Environmental Risk Factors (BCERF)

This Web site is a resource that provides science-based information on the relationships between breast cancer and environmental risk factors, including pesticides and dietary factors. The materials were developed for a diverse audience, including consumers, educators, public policymakers, scientists, and media representatives.
World Wide Web URL: http://cfe.cornell.edu/bcerf/

National Alliance of Breast Cancer Organizations

Resources, access to clinical trials, help groups, links, and up-coming events are all offered at this site.
World Wide Web URL: http://www.nabco.org/

Cancer

Art BeCAUSE

An on-line source for greeting cards designed for cancer patients. This offering is a collection of cards expressing love and support. The majority of the cards carry empowering messages appropriate for a wide range of different life events, including, but not limited to, coping with serious illness. All cards are blank inside. A percentage of proceeds from sales is donated to research and organizations committed to ending breast cancer.
World Wide Web URL: http://www.electricmedia.com/web/artbecause

Breast Cancer Information Clearinghouse

A repository for current information about breast cancer funded by the New York State Science and Technology Foundation (NYSERNet). NYSERNet, Inc. established the Breast Cancer Information Clearinghouse in 1994 at a time when there was little or no useful content on the Internet for a breast cancer patient. The BCIC was formed as a partnership of local and national organizations dedicated to the fight of this disease. These organizations provided the content for the site, and NYSERNet provided the tools and technology necessary to make this information available to the world.
World Wide Web URL: http://www.nabco.org/resources/

Breast Cancer Roundtable

This site is devoted to issues concerning breast cancer, and contains information from many on-line journals, research studies, and organizations. A new issue will be presented each month. Your opinion may be inputted.
World Wide Web URL: http://www.seas.gwu.edu/student/tlooms/ MGT243/bcr.html

Canadian Cancer Society

The leading Canadian nonprofit organization focusing on education about cancer prevention and treatment.
World Wide Web URL: http://www.cancer.ca

Cancer Information from the International Cancer Alliance

This new home page presents ICA's highly successful cancer information program. Its approach provides a source of continuing patient-driven information (on 42 types of adult and pediatric cancers) for patients, their families, and their physicians. ICA has developed these programs through the International Cancer Academy for Research and Education (ICARE). The ICARE organization is a network of people: scientists, caring staff, and lay volunteers. This network provides information and interaction with world-class scientists, doctors, and lay persons—all united in the quest to conquer or at least deal effectively with cancer.
World Wide Web URL: http://www.icare.org/index.htm

CancerGuide: Steve Dunn's Cancer Information Page

CancerGuide is dedicated to helping consumers find the answers to their questions about cancer, and especially to helping patients find the questions they need to ask.
World Wide Web URL: http://cancerguide.org/

CancerNet

The National Cancer Institute's CancerNet service makes the cancer information statements from PDQ and other cancer information from the NCI available quickly and easily via the Internet and selected other electronic information services.
World Wide Web URL: http://cancernet.nci.nih.gov/

Leukaemia Research Fund Home Page

The Leukaemia Research Fund is the only United Kingdom research charity devoted to research into the causes, treatment, and prevention of leukemia and related diseases. The site covers all forms of leukemia and lymphoma, multiple myeloma, myelodysplastic syndromes, myeloproliferative disorders, and aplastic anemia.
World Wide Web URL: http://www.leukaemia-research.org.uk

National Alliance of Breast Cancer Organizations

Resources, access to clinical trials, help groups, links, and up-coming events are all offered at this site.
World Wide Web URL: http://www.nabco.org/

National Cancer Institute

Home page for the National Cancer Institute.
World Wide Web URL: http://www.nci.nih.gov/

National Cancer Institute

News and abstracts from the *Journal of the National Cancer Institute* (JNCI) and other NCI publications. Connect with CANCERLIT, a comprehensive archival file of more than 1,000,000 bibliographic records describing cancer results published for the past 30 years in biomedical journals, proceedings of scientific meetings, books, technical reports, and other documents.
World Wide Web URL: http://www.nci.nih.gov

National Cervical Cancer Coalition

The coalition enhances awareness of the traditional Pap smear, new technologies, and reimbursement issues facing cervical cancer screening. The site offers information about research, early detection, reimbursement, and general patient information.
World Wide Web URL: http://www.nccc-online.org/

Prostate Cancer Home Page

The University of Michigan Prostate Cancer Home Page is designed to provide prostate cancer-related information pertaining to diagnosis, staging, treatment options, specialists, investigational studies, and current research. A forum for

e-mail communication is provided. It is intended for health professionals and interested patients alike.
World Wide Web URL: http://www.cancer.med.umich.edu/prostcan/ prostcan.html

Society of Gynecologic Oncologists

Here you will find an introduction to the specialty of gynecologic oncology and information about gynecological cancers from the SGO.
World Wide Web URL: http://www.sgo.org/

The Testicular Cancer Research Center

This site manages to tastefully add a humorous side to the most common cancer in males ages 15 to 35. Contains the long and short of testicular cancer, personal stories, treatment options, and more.
World Wide Web URL: http://www.acor.org/diseases/TC/

Children's Health Issues

BabyCenter

Packed full of advice and info for expectant and new parents, covering every conceivable topic to do with pregnancy, babies, and family life.
World Wide Web URL: http://www.babycenter.com/

Children's Medical Center of Dallas

Home page for the Children's Medical Center of Dallas.
World Wide Web URL: http://www.childrens.com/

Infectious Diseases in Children

Infectious Diseases in Children provides news and information to help medical professionals who take care of children. This site claims to be the primary news source for pediatricians, covering new drugs and procedures for diagnosing and testing pediatric infectious diseases. This monthly newspaper presents succinct reports from medical symposia, as well as interviews with the experts in pediatric infectious diseases, keeping pediatricians aware of current developments in diagnostic practices and procedures, vaccines, drugs, and treatment. Physicians can apply this information to their daily practice.
World Wide Web URL: http://www.slackinc.com/child/idc/idchome.htm

KidsHealth

Comprehensive site for kids and parents covering issues such as growth, food and fitness, childhood infections, and immunization. Created by the Alfred I. duPont Hospital for Children, the Nemours Children's Clinics.
World Wide Web URL: http://KidsHealth.org/

MedConnect

MedConnect provides educational services to emergency and primary care physicians and pediatricians, CME, interesting cases, board reviews, and chest radiology teaching file.
World Wide Web URL: http://www.medconnect.com/

Pedinfo

Information for pediatricians, parents, and others interested in child health. The site includes an extensive list of links.
World Wide Web URL: http://www.pedinfo.org/

The Wonderful Worlds of Internal Medicine and Pediatriacs

A series of links and lists dealing with issues revolving around internal medicine and pediatrics individually and as a combined specialty.
World Wide Web URL: http://ourworld.compuserve.com/homepages/ anduril/medicin2.htm

Communicable Disease

CDC Emerging Infectious Disease Journal

The journal *Emerging Infectious Diseases*, published by the National Center for Infectious Diseases, Centers for Disease Control and Prevention, tracks trends and provides synthesis and analysis of new and reemerging infectious disease issues around the world. The publisher welcomes articles from all disciplines whose study elucidates the factors influencing the emergence and reemergence of infectious diseases.
World Wide Web URL: http://www.cdc.gov/ncidod/eid/index.htm

Infectious Diseases Society of America

The Infectious Diseases Society of America is an organization of physicians, scientists, and other health care professionals dedicated to promoting human

health through excellence in research,education, prevention, and care of patients. The society pursues and represents the concerns of its membership by its organizational structure, journals, meetings, and other activities. The site contains links and information about meetings, job opportunities, and links to other sites.
World Wide Web URL: http://www.idsociety.org/

Prevention News Update database

The Prevention News Update databases contains over 26,000 abstracts of articles about HIV/AIDS-, STD-, and TB-related events in the news; trends in these epidemics; and research findings from major newspapers, wire services, medical journals, and news magazines.
World Wide Web URL: http://www.cdcnpin.org/db/public/dnmain.htm

Public Health Laboratory Service

The Public Health Laboratory Service (PHLS) of England and Wales is a national network comprising public health laboratories, reference laboratories, and the Communicable Disease Surveillance Centre. The Communicable Disease Surveillance Centre (CDSC) was established in 1977 to undertake national surveillance of communicable disease and to provide epidemiological assistance and coordination in the investigation and control of infection in England and in Wales.
World Wide Web URL: http://www.phls.co.uk/

Travel Health Online

An on-line site that provides information about travel related health issues.
World Wide Web URL: http://www.tripprep.com

Computers and Health

ACP Online Computers and Medicine

Past articles from the ACP Observer by the American College of Physicians (ACP) concerning computers and medicine and their integration.
World Wide Web URL: http://www.acponline.org/journals/news/ compmed.htm

Depression

DMDA Depression Site

The DMDA of Mount Sinai Medical Center is a support group for persons with mood disorders, depression, and bipolar disorder, as well as their family members and friends.
World Wide Web URL: http://www.columbia.edu/~jgg17/DMDA/

National Depressive and Manic-Depressive Association

The mission of the National Depressive and Manic-Depressive Association is to educate patients, families, professionals, and the public concerning the nature of depressive and manic-depressive illness as treatable medical diseases; to foster self-help for patients and families; to eliminate discrimination and stigma; to improve access to care; and to advocate for research toward the elimination of these illnesses. This site attempts to fulfill this mission through information and links.
World Wide Web URL: http://www.ndmda.org/

Dermatology

AMA Archives of Dermatology

The site offers information about the *Archives of Dermatology*, an opportunity to register to get the table of contents via e-mail, and current or past tables of contents.
World Wide Web URL: http://www.ama-assn.org/public/journals/derm/ dermhome.htm

American Academy of Dermatology

Info on the AAD, plus public information on dermatology, research, and news. The site allows you to search for a dermatologist near you.
World Wide Web URL: http://www.aad.org/

Dermatology On-line Journal

Visit this site for recent articles, proceedings, and announcements regarding dermatology.
World Wide Web URL: http://dermatology.cdlib.org/DOJvol1num1/ journal.html

Dermatology Times

A newspaper-format publication for the field of dermatology.
World Wide Web URL: http://www.dermatologytimes.com/

DermDigest—The On-line Dermatology Conference

Information, on-line interactions, skin care tips, and regular columns make up
this interesting site.
World Wide Web URL: http://dermdigest.com/

SkinCarePhysicians.com

This Web site provides patients with up-to-date information on the treatment
and management of disorders of the skin, hair, and nails. Patients and health care
professionals may utilize this Web site as a resource for educational literature
and health guideline descriptions. Information on specific disorders is sponsored
and codeveloped with industry and the medical community.
World Wide Web URL: http://www.derm-infonet.com/

Diabetes

Canadian Diabetes Association

The Canadian Diabetes Association's Internet site is another way to fulfill its
mission of promoting the health of Canadians through diabetes research, service,
education, and advocacy. The CDA's site provides information about the
association along with informative and up-to-the-minute articles. The contents
range from medical position papers suitable for researchers and physicians interested in diabetes to articles for those who are just learning to live with the
disease.
World Wide Web URL: http://www.diabetes.ca/

Children with Diabetes

A site dedicated to patients and parents of children with childhood diabetes.
**World Wide Web URL: http://www.childrenwithdiabetes.com/
index_cwd.htm**

Diabetes Interview

The mission statement of this site is to provide current and accurate information on diabetes and its care. Its goal is for all people with diabetes to lead healthy and fulfilling lives.
World Wide Web URL: http://www.diabetesworld.com/

Diabetes Monitor

This site monitors diabetes happenings "everywhere in cyberspace." A wide-ranging list of Web pages about various aspects of diabetes care, subdivided by topic. A "hodgepodge" of hyperlinks to huge and humble home pages, Web sites, and Web pages that have information about diabetes and related health issues.
World Wide Web URL: http://www.mdcc.com

Juvenile Diabetes Foundation

The Juvenile Diabetes Foundation is a not-for-profit, voluntary health agency whose mission is to support and fund research to find a cure for diabetes and its complications.
World Wide Web URL: http://www.jdrf.org/

Managing Your Diabetes

Diabetes information for health care professionals, patients, and consumers in the U.S. including a what's new section, diabetes news and events, education center, questions and answers, medical issues, diabetes games, as well as information regarding a pilot program.
World Wide Web URL: http://www.lillydiabetes.com/

National Institute of Diabetes and Digestive and Kidney Diseases

This is the Web site for the National Institute of Diabetes and Digestive and Kidney Diseases of the National Institutes of Health. Providing information for the public, patients, health educators, and health care providers about diabetes, digestive diseases, endocrine diseases, hematologic diseases, kidney diseases, nutrition and obesity, and urologic diseases.
World Wide Web URL: http://www.niddk.nih.gov/

On-line Resources for Diabetics

Like just about everything else on the Internet and the rest of on-line space, support and information resources for diabetics are fragmented and hard to find.

This FAQ is an attempt to bring together in one place a directory of all those places where diabetics can find what is available.
World Wide Web URL: http://www.mendosa.com/faq.htm

Diet and Nutrition

2000 Calories a Day

Includes daily meal planner, menu ideas, recipes, and calorie/fat analysis.
World Wide Web URL: http://www.caloriecontrol.org/recipes.html

American Dietetic Association

Information about up-coming meetings, the society's journal, and portals to a wealth of information on nutrition and diet can be found at this site.
World Wide Web URL: http://www.eatright.org

National Network for Child Care: Nutrition

Articles about family nutrition including advice on feeding infants, pesticides in food, and kid's snacks. The site also contains a guide to children's weight.
World Wide Web URL: http://www.nncc.org/Nutrition/nutr.page.html

Weight Watchers International

Searchable database of meetings in North America, with information about their programs, food products, and how to join.
World Wide Web URL: http://www.weight-watchers.com/

Digestive Disease

American Gastroenterological Association

Home page for the American Gastroenterological Association.
World Wide Web URL: http://www.gastro.org/

National Institute of Diabetes and Digestive and Kidney Diseases (of the NIH)

This is the official home page of the National Institute of Diabetes and Digestive and Kidney Diseases (NIDDK) of the National Institutes of Health (NIH). The National Institute of Diabetes and Digestive and Kidney Diseases conducts and

supports research on many of the most serious diseases affecting public health. The institute supports much of the clinical research on the diseases of internal medicine and related subspecialty fields as well as many basic science disciplines. The site provides access to much of this material for patients and practitioners alike.
World Wide Web URL: http://www.niddk.nih.gov/

Endocrine Disorders

HealthWeb:Endocrinology

This page is a collaborative effort of the Northwestern University Galter Health Sciences Library and the HealthWeb project. HealthWeb is a cooperative initiative of the health sciences libraries of the Committee on Institutional Cooperation (CIC) and the National Network of Libraries of Medicine Greater Midwest Region.
World Wide Web URL: http://www.galter.nwu.edu/hw/endo/

National Institute of Diabetes and Digestive and Kidney Diseases

This is the Web site for National Institute of Diabetes and Digestive and Kidney Diseases of the National Institutes of Health. Providing information for the public, patients, health educators, and health care providers about diabetes, digestive diseases, endocrine diseases, hematologic diseases, kidney diseases, nutrition and obesity, and urologic diseases.
World Wide Web URL: http://www.niddk.nih.gov/

Society for Endocrinology

The Society for Endocrinology aims to promote the advancement of public education in endocrinology.
World Wide Web URL: http://www.endocrinology.org/

Epilepsy

Epilepsy Foundation of America Home Page

This site offers the usual information about the foundation and its services, along with disease-specific information for patients. Unique aspects of this site, however, are a kids club and teen chat room.
World Wide Web URL: http://www.efa.org/

FAQ—Epilepsy

Frequently asked questions (and answers) about Epilepsy.
World Wide Web URL: http://debra.dgbt.doc.ca/~andrew/epilepsy/

Ethics

American Society for Bioethics and Humanities (ASBH)

Provides information about the American Society for Bioethics and Humanities (ASBH). It is a professional society of more than 1,200 individuals, organizations, and institutions interested in bioethics and humanities. This Web site, established in January 1998, is intended initially to serve as a source of information about ASBH for members and prospective members. It also will serve as a resource for anyone interested in bioethics and humanities by providing a group of further on-line resources and links to aid in finding other related information through the Internet.
World Wide Web URL: http://www.asbh.org/

Human Subjects and Research Ethics

This page is intended to provide pointers to information about ethical aspects of research involving human subjects as participants.
World Wide Web URL: http://www.psych.bangor.ac.uk/deptpsych/Ethics/ HumanResearch.html

National Reference Center for Bioethics Literature

The National Reference Center for Bioethics Literature offers specialized collection of books, journals, and other documents concerned with ethical issues in medicine and the professions, especially contemporary biomedical issues.
World Wide Web URL: http://www.georgetown.edu/research/nrcbl/

Fitness and Exercise

The Fitness Jumpsite

A Web site that proclaims that it wants to be "your connection to a lifestyle of fitness, nutrition and health." It contains information and links to fitness and lifestyle issues. A great little grass roots site (read: non commercial labor of love) providing extensive links and content for the fitness-minded, along with support for people struggling to lose weight or otherwise get in shape. This

everything-to-everyone resource also lets you investigate a new sport, search reviews of sports equipment, or browse hundreds of links to other Web sites.
World Wide Web URL: http://www.primusweb.com/fitnesspartner/

Fitness Online

Cool site with advice on fitness, training, and nutrition. Provides links to 'zines including *Shape, Muscle and Fitness, Flex,* and *Men's Fitness.*
World Wide Web URL: http://www.fitnessonline.com/

Shape Up America!

Designed to provide the latest information about safe weight management and physical fitness. The site includes keyword and concept searches.
World Wide Web URL: http://www.shapeup.org/

Gynecology and Women's Health

A Forum for Women's Health

A Forum for Women's Health, sponsored by Healthwire, features "Ask A Woman Doctor," life-cycle information, and the ability to do subject searches. The site's host, Healthwire, is a forum through which commercial, nonprofit, and grass roots organizations provide information to the general and professional public regarding various health issues
World Wide Web URL: http://www.womenshealth.org

American College of Nurse-Midwives

Contains information about nurse-midwifery practice, how to find nurse-midwives, ACNM chapters, nurse-midwifery education programs, and the ACNM news journal, *Quickening.*
World Wide Web URL: http://www.acnm.org/

Ask NOAH about Pregnancy

Ask NOAH about Pregnancy is almost, but not quite, an FAQ for pregnancy. Also links to other resources.
World Wide Web URL: http://www.noah-health.org/english/pregnancy/ pregnancy.html

Birthcontrol.com

A British site that provides information on a large selection of birth control and women's health products that are available nowhere else. Just move your mouse over any flower on the opening page to get started with information about these products. This site provides an interesting look at birth control and commerce in other parts of the world. Most of the items for sale are not approved in the United States.
World Wide Web URL: http://www.birthcontrol.com/

Breast-Feeding Resources

Rresources for breast-feeding, new and expectant parents. Provides a group of links to other sites as well.
World Wide Web URL: http://users.aol.com/kristachan/brstres.htm

Childbirth.org

An alternative-birth information service that provides information for consumers.
World Wide Web URL: http://www.childbirth.org/index.html

Eve's Apple

Humorous site with reviews and articles.
World Wide Web URL: http://www.evesapple.com/

Femina: Web Search for Women

Provides a searchable directory of links to female friendly sites on the Web. It offers links for information on violence, sexuality, and fitness.
World Wide Web URL: http://femina.cybergrrl.com/

Findings: The Women's Health Care Advocacy Service

Encouraging women to make thoughtful choices about their health by providing them with information and support.
World Wide Web URL: http://www.findings.net

Gynecologic Oncology Tutorials at the University of Washington

These tutorials were prepared with the junior and senior residents in mind by the Division of Gynecologic Oncology, University of Washington. It has tutorials

for teaching purposes designed to supplement currently available learning resources.
World Wide Web URL: http://gynoncology.obgyn.washington.edu/

Healthtouch: Birth Control

A group of links and information pages about birth control issues.
World Wide Web URL: http://www.healthtouch.com

Jacobs Institute of Women's Health

Jacobs identifies and studies women's health care issues involving the interaction of medical and social systems, and facilitates dialogue and fosters awareness among consumers and providers. The site offers publications, and conference and current events information.
World Wide Web URL: http://www.jiwh.org/

Menopause: Another Change in Life

Menopause: Another Change in Life provides resources from Planned Parenthood, including signs and indications, osteoporosis, and traditional and alternative therapies.
World Wide Web URL: http://www.plannedparenthood.org

Museum of Menstruation

The home page of the only museum in the world devoted to menstruation! The purpose of the museum is to teach the public the rich history of menstruation from all cultures of the world, and give researchers access to its unmatched collections.
World Wide Web URL: http://www.mum.org/

National Cervical Cancer Coalition

The coalition enhances awareness of the traditional Pap smear, new technologies, and reimbursement issues facing cervical cancer screening. The site offers information about research, early detection, and reimbursement, and general patient information.
World Wide Web URL: http://www.nccc-online.org/

National Osteoporosis Foundation

Learn about osteoporosis, a key concern for women in their menopausal years, at this site.
World Wide Web URL: http://www.nof.org

National Women's Health Resource Center

Quite possibly the leading U.S. federal clearinghouse for women's health information.
World Wide Web URL: http://www.healthywomen.org/

North American Menopause Society

The NAMS Web site deals with issues about menopause, including information about the society. It contains information, publications, and links related to menopause.
World Wide Web URL: http://www.menopause.org/

OBGYN.net

This is a physician-reviewed service offering medical professionals, women, and industry a home for publishing, accessing information, and global interaction. It offers three sections, each focusing on different segments of the women's health community: medical professionals, medical industry, and women. The site contains comprehensive resources for women and health professionals. It features advice about gynecological conditions, pregnancy, news, and chat.
World Wide Web URL: obgyn.net/

Online Birth Center

Midwifery, pregnancy and birth-related information.
World Wide Web URL: http://www.moonlily.com/obc/

Planned Parenthood Federation of America

Looking for resources on sexual and reproductive health, family planning, STDs, or sexuality education? The home page for Planned Parenthood includes education resources for a variety of audiences on these topics, and more, as well as extensive links to related organizations. The site offers a Spanish-language option as well.
World Wide Web URL: http://www.plannedparenthood.org/

PMS Center

PMS Center offers descriptions and symptoms: psychological, postpartum depression, learning disabilities, etc., associated with premenstrual syndromes.
World Wide Web URL: http://www.bairpms.com/

Pregnancy Related E-mail Lists

Pregnancy Related E-mail Lists include the ICAN on-line cesarean support group, midwife, doula, childbirth educators, and apprentice midwife lists.
World Wide Web URL: http://www.fensende.com

Pregnancy at Women.com

Interactive pregnancy/childbirth resource center with weekly description of your baby/pregancy changes, chat rooms, bulletin board, and more. It includes a section of "underbellies"—a collection of personal glimpses of the ups and downs of pregnancy and nursing.
World Wide Web URL: http://www.women.com/pregnancy/

ProMoM

What you can do to support breast-feeding in your community. How to find help and information about breast-feeding.
World Wide Web URL: http://www.promom.org

Society of Gynecologic Oncologists

Here you will find an introduction to the specialty of gynecologic oncology and information about gynecological cancers from the SGO.
World Wide Web URL: http://www.sgo.org/

Tampax

Facts on menopause, its symptoms, hormone replacement therapy, depression, sexuality, and more, are accessible via the Tampax site. The site is useful for parents with teenage daughters.
World Wide Web URL: http://www.tampax.com

The Universe of Women's Health

A physician-reviewed service offering medical professionals, women, and industry a home for publishing, accessing information, and global interaction. It

offers three sections, each focusing on different segments of the women's health community: medical professionals, medical industry, and women.
World Wide Web URL: http://www.obgyn.net/

Waterbirth Information

The Waterbirth Web site, provides in-depth information on the use of water for labor, childbirth, and early childhood development. Includes fascinating information from the world's leading water birth pioneers, product information, and a photo gallery (including birth and breast-feeding-under-water photos).
World Wide Web URL: http://www.waterbirthinfo.com

Women's Health Interactive

Women's Health Interactive's mission is to create a learning environment where multidisciplinary health education resources are accessible to women and health care professionals. The National Women's Health Resource Center provides the site with "What's Hot in Women's Health!"—health updates from its award-winning publication, the National Women's Health Report.
World Wide Web URL: http://www.womens-health.com

Headache

American Council for Headache Education (ACHE)

American Council for Headache Education (ACHE, a national nonprofit patient/ physician partnership) site provides education, information, and support for headache suffers and their families in accordance with their goal of educating the public about this common, sometimes disabling pain disorder. Headache sufferers and their families can find education and support from the ACHE.
World Wide Web URL: http://www.achenet.org/

Migraine Relief Center

The Migraine Resource Center examines the triggers, symptoms, and treatment programs available for migraines. Free diagnostic screenings, support materials, and subscriptions to HeadWay are available. Here you can learn about some of the triggers, symptoms, and treatment programs for migraine, take a free detailed diagnostic screening, receive complimentary support materials such as a free subscription to HeadWay, the migraine newsletter, and much more. Maintained by Glaxo Wellcome, Inc.
World Wide Web URL: http://www.migrainehelp.com

National Headache Foundation

The NHF offers topic sheets and educational materials about headaches and migraines.
World Wide Web URL: http://www.headaches.org

The unOfficial Migraine Foundation Home Page

The Migraine Foundation is dedicated to serving the needs of more than 3 million Canadians suffering from migraine through awareness and educational activities. This unofficial page was created for demonstration purposes only and has not been endorsed by the Migraine Foundation. The site is temporarily offline due to a lack of funds, but may be back up and running by the time of publication.
World Wide Web URL: http://www.niagara.com/migraine/

Health Promotion and Wellness

Agency for Health Care Policy and Research

A portal to a wide range of health-related topics and literature made available by the Agency for Health Care Policy and Research.
World Wide Web URL: http://www.ahcpr.gov/clinic/

American Red Cross

Access to information and services provided by the American Red Cross including health education, health services, blood services, and disaster relief. The site also hosts an extensive "virtual museum" with images and information about the history and development of the American Red Cross.
World Wide Web URL: http://www.redcross.org

Black Health Net

An on-line source for information on health issues important to African Americans. Users may submit anonymous questions or search the database of topics offered.
World Wide Web URL: http://www.blackhealthnetwork.com/

Center for Science in the Public Interest

Looking for information on nutrition for adults and kids, olestra, or alcohol? The CSPI provides it here and in its Nutrition Action Newsletter. You'll also find links to other nutrition sites.
World Wide Web URL: http://www.cspinet.org

The Daily Apple

Medical health guide full of news and advice. Find resources on illness, disease prevention, lifestyle, family, and everyday health.
World Wide Web URL: http://thedailyapple.com/

Femina: Web Search for Women

Provides a searchable directory of links to female-friendly sites on the Web. It offers links for information on violence, sexuality, and fitness.
World Wide Web URL: http://femina.cybergrrl.com/

Fitness Partnet Connection Jumpsite

A great little grass-roots site (read: noncommercial labor of love) providing extensive links and content for the fitness-minded, along with support for people struggling to lose weight or otherwise get in shape. This everything-to-everyone resource also lets you investigate a new sport, search reviews of sports equipment, or browse hundreds of links to other Web sites.
World Wide Web URL: http://www.primusweb.com/fitnesspartner/

FitnessZone's Fitness Profile

Easy-to-complete fitness assessment that helps calculate your target workout heart rate, and gives advice on general fitness goals. It provides you with a detailed fitness profile, including overall fitness rating and nutrition and exercise plans, and recommends a pace for you to exercise, based on this profile.
World Wide Web URL: http://www.fitnesszone.com/profiles/

Guide to Clinical Preventive Services: Second Edition (1996)

A full-text version of the *Guide to Clinical Preventive Services*: Second Edition. The text may be searched or downloaded for printing.
World Wide Web URL: http://text.nlm.nih.gov/ftrs/
pick?collect=cps&dbName=0&cc=1&t=909152904

The Health Mall: Health, Nutrition, Fitness, and Personal Development

The Health Mall is both a resource center and shopping mall featuring businesses that offer products, services, and information related to health, nutrition, fitness, and personal development. Some stores are strictly informational, others offer on-line ordering; some offer coupons. The mall includes a searchable database of health food stores in the U.S., an on-line magazine called "A Healthy Day," a classified section, and a resource center.
World Wide Web URL: http://www.hlthmall.com

Health Risk Assessment

Hosted by Beth Israel Medical Center, this self-assessment quiz provides simple health and fitness advice.
World Wide Web URL: http://www.bimc.edu/interactive/assessment.html

Healthcentral.com

The former Planet Health has become part of Healthcentral.com. Visit this site for a fine collection of resources and health news stories, and even do a little shopping.
World Wide Web URL: http://www.healthcentral.com/home/home.cfm

HealthWorld On-line

With a strong emphasis on alternative and complementary therapies, HealthWorld On-line provides a variety of resources on issues including nutrition, fitness, and self-care. The interface is an nice graphic representation of a small town.
World Wide Web URL: http://www.healthy.net

InteliHealth—Johns Hopkins

Features daily news articles, health quizzes, ask-the-doc, health library, and loads of informative health information.
World Wide Web URL: http://www.intellihealth.com/IH/ihtIH

OBGYN.net

This is a physician-reviewed service offering medical professionals, women, and industry a home for publishing, accessing information, and global interaction. It offers three sections, each focusing on different segments of the women's health community: medical professionals, medical industry, and women. The site con-

tains comprehensive resources for women and health professionals. It features advice about gynecological conditions, pregnancy, news, and chat.
World Wide Web URL: http://www.obgyn.net/

Prevention News Update Database

The Prevention News Update databases contains over 26,000 abstracts of articles about HIV/AIDS-, STD-, and TB-related events in the news; trends in these epidemics; and research findings from major newspapers, wire services, medical journals, and news magazines.
World Wide Web URL: http://www.cdcnpin.org/db/public/dnmain.htm

U. C. Davis Wellness Center

A general guide to health and health promotion aimed at patients and provided by the University of California at Davis.
World Wide Web URL: http://wellness.ucdavis.edu/

Wellness Web

Wellness Web addresses a wide range of illnesses and diseases and caters to the information and support needs of patients.
World Wide Web URL: http://www.wellweb.com

Women's Health Interactive

Women's Health Interactive's mission is to create a learning environment where multidisciplinary health education resources are accessible to women and health care professionals. The National Women's Health Resource Center provides the site with "What's Hot in Women's Health!"—health updates from its award-winning publication, the *National Women's Health Report*.
World Wide Web URL: http://www.womens-health.com

Worldguide: Health and Fitness

Worldguide addresses human anatomy, strength training, cardiovascular exercise, eating, and sports medicine.
World Wide Web URL: http://www.worldguide.com/Fitness/hf.html

Your Health

A general compilation of information and links to further information and organizations.
World Wide Web URL: http://www.yourhealth.com/

Heart Disease

Adult Echocardiography @Columbia-Presbyterian Medical Center

This site offers a series of images in echocardiography. Two formats are available to view images. A question and answer method allows physicians and ultrasound technologists to test themselves. The library allows the individual to view images based on the diagnosis.
World Wide Web URL: http://cpmcnet.columbia.edu:80/dept/cardiology/echo/

American Heart Association

The official home page of the American Heart Association is filled with lots of information for consumers and health professionals, with links to other sources.
World Wide Web URL: http://www.americanheart.org

Cardiology Compass

A guide to cardiology information and sites provided by the Washington University School of Medicine.
World Wide Web URL: http://cardiologycompass.com

Cardiovascular Institute of the South

The Cardiovascular Institute of the South presents for education and republication a wide-ranging library of doctor column-style reports on heart disease.
World Wide Web URL: http://www.cardio.com/

Heart Information Network

A site founded by a heart patient and physician that provides news and information about heart disease.
World Wide Web URL: http://www.heartinfo.org/

Heart Surgery Forum

The Heart Surgery Forum (HSF) is an information center for the electronic distribution of manuscripts, abstracts, commentary, and other developments in the field of cardiac surgery. The forum was established to improve the distribution of new ideas, discoveries, surgical techniques, and pertinent data from all sources, both academic and nonacademic.
World Wide Web URL: http://www.hsforum.com/

Heart Surgery On-line

An eclectic site best described in its own words: "JOIN ME, and we will explore this wonderful organ.... Discover the complexities of its structure.... Journey down the blood stream and experience the efficiency of the circulation.... See how diseases of the heart are detected.... Marvel at the miracle that is 'Open Heart Surgery'.... Learn about the people who make it happen.... Understand all about the different birth defects of the heart, and how they are repaired."
**World Wide Web URL: http://www.geocities.com/HotSprings/1652/
heartintro.html**

Mental Health

American Psychological Association

This is the Internet service of the American Psychological Association. It has a great deal of material for the public and APA members. "What You Should Know about Women and Depression" is just one of the valuable articles available at the APA site.
World Wide Web URL: http://www.apa.org/

Internet Mental Health

Internet Mental Health is a free encyclopedia of mental health information.
World Wide Web URL: http://www.mentalhealth.com/p.html

Knowledge Exchange Network (KEN)

Knowledge Exchange Network (KEN) is a one-stop source of information and resources on prevention, treatment, and rehabilitation services for mental illness. KEN is a service of the Center for Mental Health Services, Substance Abuse and Mental Health Services Administration, U.S. Department of Health and Human Services. KEN offers information related to consumers/survivors, managed care, children's mental health, statistics, and upcoming conferences and events. KEN offers an on-line database lookup of mental health resources around the country and in the local community.
World Wide Web URL: http://www.mentalhealth.org/

National Institute of Mental Health

Information on specific mental disorders, diagnosis and treatment, mental illness in America, consensus conference proceedings, NIMH long-range plans and research reports, publications order forms, quicktime videos, information on the DEPRESSION Awareness, Recognition, and Treatment (D/ART) and the Anxi-

ety Disorders Education Program, and other resources. Press advisories, press office information, listing of mental health meetings and conferences through 1998, and announcements and agendas for some upcoming conferences and meetings are also included.
World Wide Web URL: http://www.nimh.nih.gov/

National Mental Health Association

Facts, figures, and discussions about mental illness in the family, depression, schizophrenia, anxiety disorders, and more are provided here by the NMHA.
World Wide Web URL: http://www.nmha.org

Men's Health

American Prostate Society

The APS created this comprehensive site where you can find general information on prostate cancer, back issues of their newsletter, "The Update," and information on becoming a member.
World Wide Web URL: http://www.ameripros.org/

Bald Man's Home Page

Comprehensive site for the follicly impaired. If you're not bald yet, you might be after searching through all this site has to offer.
World Wide Web URL: http://www.thebaldman.com/

Health News and Information Directory

Comprehensive resource of men's health-related topics indexed by medical condition. Gives current news on the condition or illness and provides links to further information.
World Wide Web URL: http://www.healthnewsdirectory.com/HealthNews/ Directory/Default.asp?Reference=HealthNews%2ECategories%3A0% 2ECategories%3A111

Impotence

Authorative information about impotence from the National Kidney and Urologic Diseases Information Clearinghouse.
World Wide Web URL: http://www.healthtouch.com/bin/EContent_HT/ hdShowLfts.asp?lftname=KIDNE088&cid=HTHLTH

Male Health Center

A wide variety of information regarding many aspects of the male species.
World Wide Web URL: http://www.malehealthcenter.com/

MEDic Men's Health Issues

Info and research on various men's health issues.
World Wide Web URL: http://medic.med.uth.tmc.edu/ptnt/00000391.htm

National Institutes of Health Consensus Development Conference Statement

Site containing articles relating to the causes of and treatments for impotence.
World Wide Web URL: http://text.nlm.nih.gov/nih/cdc/www/91txt.html

Prostate Pointers

A full spectrum of information about prostate cancer and general problems of the prostate.
World Wide Web URL: http://prostatepointers.org/prostate/

Successfully Treating Impotence

This site offers information on the incidence and causes of impotence. It also dispels myths, reveals facts, and offers hope to impotence sufferers.
World Wide Web URL: http://www.impotent.com/

Testicular Cancer Research Center

This site manages to tastefully add a humorous side to the most common cancer in males ages 15 to 35. Contains the long and short of testicular cancer, personal stories, treatment options, and more.
World Wide Web URL: http://www.acor.org/diseases/TC/

Occupational Health

Canada's National Occupational Health and Safety Web Page

"The purpose of this site is to enable Canadians to easily and independently locate occupational health and safety information for the purpose of legal compliance, improving workplace health and safety practices, and ultimately to

facilitate the acquisition of information required for reduction in workplace injuries and illnesses, by providing Canadians with a convenient, single location on the Internet to access the health and safety information provided by the federal, provincial, and territorial governments of Canada and by the Canadian Centre for Occupational Health and Safety." (The preceding was supplied verbatim by the Canadian Government. Who says governments can't say things in a simple manner?)
World Wide Web URL: http://www.ccohs.ca/natosh/oshdefault.html

Canadian Centre for Occupational Health and Safety

The Canadian Centre for Occupational Health and Safety (CCOHS) promotes a safe and healthy working environment by providing information and advice about occupational health and safety.
World Wide Web URL: http://www.msds.org/

Environmental and Occupational Health Resource Guide

The Environmental and Occupational Health Sciences Institute (EOHSI) compiled the environmental and occupational health resource guide to help the media, industry, and government find the experts they need when addressing issues involving environmental and occupational health. The first issue was met with such success in 1995 that it was decided to update the guide annually to include new members and areas of expertise.
World Wide Web URL: http://www.eohsi.rutgers.edu/guide.html

Repetitive Strain Injury Primer

The Computer-Related Repetitive Strain Injury page informs computer users of their risk of physical injury. In brief format, it discusses what RSI is, major symptoms, prevention measures, what to do if symptoms already exist, and where to learn more about RSI through a book and Web site list.
World Wide Web URL: http://www.engr.unl.edu/ee/eeshop/rsi.html

Renal, Kidney, and Urinary Tract Disease

General Information about Interstitial Cystitis (IC)

All you ever wanted to know about interstitial cystitis.
World Wide Web URL: http://www.healthtouch.com/bin/EContent_HT/ hdSubIndex.asp?goto_type=1x5-Grid&index=120645&title=Interstitial+ Cystitis&cid=HTHLTH

National Institute of Diabetes and Digestive and Kidney Diseases

This is the Web site for the National Institute of Diabetes and Digestive and Kidney Diseases of the National Institutes of Health. Providing information for the public, patients, health educators, and health care providers about diabetes, digestive diseases, endocrine diseases, hematologic diseases, kidney diseases, nutrition and obesity, and urologic diseases.
World Wide Web URL: http://www.niddk.nih.gov/

Sexuality and Sexual Dysfunction

Ask NOAH about: Sexuality

New York Online Access to Health (NOAH) is a project that brought together four New York partners: the City University of New York, the New York Academy of Medicine, New York Metropolitan Reference and Research Library Agency, and the New York Public Libary. This site provides a number of FAQs about sexuality and sex-related issues.
World Wide Web URL: http://www.noah-health.org/english/sexuality/ sexuality.html

Coalition for Positive Sexuality Resources

A list of Web and telephone resources on sex and sexuality topics.
World Wide Web URL: http://www.positive.org/%7Ecps/Home/index.html

Complete Internet Sex Resource Guide

A guide and links resource. (The site contains content suitable for those over 18.)
World Wide Web URL: http://sleepingbeauty.com/world/netsex.html

Gay/Lesbian Politics and Law

A selective, annotated guide to the best and most authoritative resources on politics, law, and policy. Designed for students, scholars, teachers, journalists, activists, and citizens, and maintained by Steve Sanders at Indiana University.
World Wide Web URL: http://www.indiana.edu/~glbtpol/

National Council on Sexual Addiction and Compulsivity (NCSAC)

Information on the existence, description, consequences, and treatments of sexual addiction.
World Wide Web URL: http://www.ncsac.org/main.html

Planned Parenthood On-line's Birth Control Information

General and specific information from Planned Parenthood.
World Wide Web URL: http://www.plannedparenthood.org/

Positive.org

Positive.org is dedicated to having a positive attitude about sexuality—gay, straight, or bi. It stresses safe sexuality and reinforces the idea that there's nothing wrong with you if you decide to have sex, and nothing wrong with you if you decide not to. The site has many topics, a glossary, and search capabilities. Site maintained by the Coalition for Positive Sexuality. (A Spanish-language version is also available.)
World Wide Web URL: http://www.positive.org/Home/index.html

Safer Sex Page

A sexual health site, the Safer Sex page offers information about birth control and safe sex. This is the largest archive of information on safe sex information on the World Wide Web.
World Wide Web URL: http://www.safersex.org/

The Sex Directory

Safe sex information and directory. A universal guide to safer sex and a directory of local (British) services.
World Wide Web URL: http://www.personal.u-net.com/~healthdv/sexweb/

Sexuality Information and Education Council of the U.S.

Nonprofit organization devoted to information about sex issues. SIECUS affirms that sexuality is a natural and healthy part of living. Incorporated in 1964, SIECUS develops, collects, and disseminates information, promotes comprehensive education about sexuality, and advocates the right of individuals to make responsible sexual choices. The site includes topics from the current news.
World Wide Web URL: http://www.siecus.org

The Society for Human Sexuality

The Society for Human Sexuality, which began as a registered student organization at the University of Washington (Seattle), is devoted to the study of human sexuality. It is a social and educational organization whose purpose is to promote understanding and appreciation for the many forms of adult intimate relationships and consensual sexual expression. This site presents information, library materials, and links about human sexuality.
World Wide Web URL: http://www.sexuality.org/

Smoking

American Lung Association

A searchable site with information about smoking and various lung diseases.
World Wide Web URL: http://www.lungusa.org/

The Ash Tray

A wide-ranging site that deals with smoking and health sponsored by the Boston University Medical Center Community Outreach Health Information System.
World Wide Web URL: http://www.bu.edu/cohis/smoking/smoke.htm

Freedom Program for Smoking Cessation

An enrollment site that offers a commercial quit smoking program.
World Wide Web URL: http://www.ucanquit.com/

Questions and Answers about Finding Smoking Cessation Services

This is the National Cancer Institute's site providing lots of information about smoking, smoking cessation, and links to useful sites. A good resource for patients (or providers) who want to quit smoking.
World Wide Web URL: http://cancernet.nci.nih.gov/clinpdq/rehab/ Questions_and_Answers_About_Finding_Smoking_Cessation_Services.html

Smoking Cessation: Helping Smokers Quit. A Guide for Primary Care Clinicians

The materials contained in the Tobacco Cessation Guideline are extensive and include audio files, text, and banners that may be used in links back to the site.

The site provides resources for health care providers including links to electronic versions of smoking cessation and and other clinical practice guidelines.
World Wide Web URL: http://www.surgeongeneral.gov/tobacco/

Pharmacy and Pharmaceuticals

Continuing Education

Health care Education and Learning Information Exchange

Helix (Health care Education Learning and Information Exchange) is a meta-health care site on the World Wide Web offering professional education and information for all health practitioners and their patients. Sponsored and managed by the Glaxo Wellcome Health care Education Department, HELIX on the World Wide Web offers point-and-click access to a wealth of health information on the Internet as well as the Web sites of a number of state and national medical, pharmacy, and nursing associations. Membership is free via on-line registration.
World Wide Web URL: http://www.HELIX.com

History and Reference

ePocrates

This Internet site makes available drug information software for the popular hand-held computers such as Palm and others. From Abelcet to Zyrtec, this proprietary database provides point-of-care information for the most commonly prescribed medications.
World Wide Web URL: http://www.epocrates.com/products/qRx/

Pharmaceuticals and Products

AstraZeneca Pharmaceuticals

An extensive site that offers news and information about the company, its products, and services.
World Wide Web URL: http://www.astrazeneca.com/

Clinical Pharmacology 2000

Search engine for commonly prescribed drugs that supplies dosages, indications, interactions, pharmacokinetics, costs, and more. This site provides chemical structures, descriptions, mechanisms of action, pharmacokinetics, indications, contraindications, drug interactions, adverse reactions, a cost index, and a classification overview. Information is available in both English and Spanish.
World Wide Web URL: http://cp.gsm.com/

Consumer Health Products Association

The Consumer Health Products Association provides information about OTC nonprescription medicines including such issues as self-care, Rx-to-OTC switch, labeling, and drug distribution. OTC facts and figures are also available.
World Wide Web URL: http://www.chpa-info.org/

Drug Formulary at Michigan Medical Center

This is an extensive drug database that includes therapeutic categories and clinical tables.
World Wide Web URL: http://www.pharm.med.umich.edu/public/

Drug InforNet

This private Health On the Net Foundation subscriber, offers a wide variety of drug-related information for both providers and patients alike. The site contains searchable databases of information taken from both the professional and patient package inserts. The information is available by brand name, generic name, manufacturer, and therapeutic class. Beyond the drug-related information supplied are links to other sites for information about diseases, medical news items, medical schools, government agencies, and hospitals.
World Wide Web URL: http://www.druginfonet.com

Glaxo Wellcome pharmaceuticals

This site provides corporate, product, and drug information. The parent company may also be accessed at: www.glaxowellcome.co.uk
World Wide Web URL: http://www.glaxowellcome.com/

Healthtouch Drug Information Search

Presents searchable information about prescriptions and over-the-counter medications including usual indications and side effects.
World Wide Web URL: http://www.healthtouch.com/level1/p_dri.htm

Infomed Drug Guide

The drugs selected for this guide represent possible staple constituents for our therapeutic arsenal. The selection does not claim to be comprehensive; in fact, it focuses on the common problems in the general practice.
World Wide Web URL: http://www.infomed.org/100drugs/

Internet FDA

The Food and Drug Administration site offers information for consumers and health professionals on a wide variety of its activities.
World Wide Web URL: http://www.fda.gov/

Martindale's Health Science Guide

This is an extensive site offering information on almost any aspect of pharmacy and pharmaceuticals.
World Wide Web URL: http://www-sci.lib.uci.edu/HSG/
Pharmacy.html#PC3

New Drugs List

A listing of new drugs, including chemical and trade names, brief description, and manufacturer.
World Wide Web URL: http://cctr.umkc.edu/user/mash/newdrugs.html

PDR for Physicians

Presented by Medical Economics (the publisher of the printed version), this site offers the *Physicians' Desk Reference* (PDR) as well as the PDR for herbal

medications and PDR for multiple drug interactions. Other options include access to new drug and pricing information.
World Wide Web URL: http://physician.pdr.net/physician/index.htm

Pfizer pharmaceuticals

Pfizer's Internet site offers the usual pharmaceutical and corporate information, but also provides links to the Mayo Clinic's Health Oasis Web site. The site offers independently authored articles that cover a broad range of medical topics from an objective, patient-oriented perspective.
World Wide Web URL: http://www.pfizer.com/main.html

Pharmacy (Medicine, Biosciences)

This page includes a number of pharmacy-related (loosely defined) Internet resources including schools of pharmacy, on-line journals, continuing education, and societies.
World Wide Web URL: http://www.cpb.uokhsc.edu/pharmacy/ pharmint.html

PharmWeb

A searchable site from the U.K. with information for the patient and health professional.
World Wide Web URL: http://www.pharmweb.net/

PhRMA

The site of the nonprofit advocacy group of the Pharmaceutical Research Manufacturers Association includes drugs in development, industry facts and figures, consumer health guides, and industry FAQs. PhRMA membership represents approximately 100 U.S. companies that have a primary commitment to pharmaceutical research.
World Wide Web URL: http://www.phrma.org

Physician's GenRX Drug Compendium Program

A comprehensive listing that is searchable by generic or brand names and by drug category.
World Wide Web URL: http://www.harcourthealth.com/Mosby/ PhyGenRx/index.html

RxList Internet Drug Name Category Cross Index

Searchable database of 4,000 prescription and OTC drug products designed for the lay public.
World Wide Web URL: http://www.rxlist.com

ScripWorld Pharmaceutical News

Scrip is the only international, twice-weekly newsletter reporting on the pharmaceutical sector, covering prescription and OTC medicines and biotechnology news.
World Wide Web URL: http://www.pjbpubs.co.uk/scrip

Top 200 Prescriptions

A list of the most commonly prescribed drugs in the U.S. This list covers the drug's action, use, contraindications, interactions, toxicity, and dosing.
World Wide Web URL: http://www.rxlist.com/top200.htm

Ancillary Support

Nursing

Delmar Publishers' Nursing Resource Center

Delmar Publishers' Nursing Resource Center including a full catalog of resources for the student, instructor, and professional. Its nursing catalog includes over 300 books and software products. On-line ordering is available as is a keyword search engine. Visitors can also browse the nursing subject areas by category.
World Wide Web URL: http://www.delmarnursing.com/

Health care Education and Learning Information Exchage

Helix (Health care Education Learning and Information Exchange) is a meta-health care site on the World Wide Web offering professional education and information for all health practitioners and their patients. Sponsored and managed by the Glaxo Wellcome Health care Education Department, HELIX on the World Wide Web offers point-and-click access to a wealth of health information on the Internet as well as the Web sites of a number of state and national medical, pharmacy, and nursing associations. Membership is free via on-line registration.
World Wide Web URL: http://www.HELIX.com

Nursing and Allied Health Jobs Site

Explore the latest health career opportunities for registered nurses and other jobs.
World Wide Web URL: http://www.health careers-online.com/ Welcome.htm

Nurse midwives

American College of Nurse-Midwives

Contains information about nurse-midwifery practice, how to find nurse-midwives, ACNM chapters, nurse-midwifery education programs, and the ACNM news journal, *Quickening*.
World Wide Web URL: http://www.acnm.org/

Childbirth.org

An alternative-birth information service that provides information for consumers.
World Wide Web URL: http://www.childbirth.org/index.html

Online Birth Center

Midwifery, pregnancy, and birth-related information.
World Wide Web URL: http://www.moonlily.com/obc/

University of Michigan Nurse—Midwifery

Information about the school, faculty, and recent graduates.
World Wide Web URL: http://sitemaker.med.umich.edu/cgi-bin/
WebObjects/sitemaker.woa/wa/displaySite?site=dswalker

Physiotherapy

American Physical Therapy Association

This site offers information for patients and physical therapists alike. Links to other Internet resources and the Amazon Books site provides additional information.
World Wide Web URL: http://www.apta.org

Respiratory Therapy

American Association of Respiratory Care

Home page for the American Association of Respiratory Care. It contains information and resources for health care professionals and AARC members.
World Wide Web URL: http://www.AARC.org

National Board of Respiratory Care

The home page for the voluntary health certifying board, which was created in
1960 to evaluate the professional competence of respiratory therapists.
World Wide Web URL: http://www.nbrc.org/

Social Work

National Association of Social Workers

A nonprofit organization for U.S. health care professionals in this specialty.
World Wide Web URL: http://www.naswdc.org

Miscellaneous

Medical News and Information

NLM National Telemedicine Initiative

This is the National Library of Medicine's site dealing with various aspects of
the National Telemedicine Initiative. There is information about the initiative,
projects supported by the initiative, up-coming meetings, and more.
World Wide Web URL: http://www.nlm.nih.gov/research/telemedinit.html

Telemedicine Information Exchange

The Telemedicine Information Exchange was created and is maintained by the
Telemedicine Research Center with major support from the National Library of
Medicine. This site is a comprehensive, international, quality-filtered resource
for information about telemedicine and telemedicine-related activities.
World Wide Web URL: http://tie.telemed.org/

Living and Lifestyle

AAA On-line

It doesn't matter if your driving needs are local, national, or international, the AAA Web site has the information you need. You can plan a trip or find out about international driver's licenses.
World Wide Web URL: http://www.aaa.com

Amazon.com

Billed as the largest on-line bookstore, it has made shopping and ordering so easy that 4.5 million customers have already bought books, music, and more. You can search for titles, subjects, or areas of interest in books, music, CDs, DVDs, and gifts. From browsing to serious shopping, with over 3 million titles, if you can't find it here you may want to rethink your needs.
World Wide Web URL: http://www.Amazon.com

At Hand Network Yellow Pages

This site is akin to an industrial-strength phone book for locating businesses.
World Wide Web URL: http://www.athand.com/

Autoweb.com

From advice on finding a new car to new car reviews and financing, this site has everything but the pushy sales people.
World Wide Web URL: http://www.autoweb.com/

Barnes and Noble Booksellers

On-line book shopping at this mega-store is easy. From just wandering about, to bargain bins, to on-line chats with current authors, the site has something for most avid bibliophiles. If you are not quite ready to do your shopping on-line, the site includes the opportunity to find the location of your nearest store by entering you zip code.
World Wide Web URL: http://www.barnesandnoble.com/

CDC Travel Information

A comprehensive guide to health-related travel information maintained by the Centers for Disease Control and Prevention. This includes information about

geographic health recommendations and current disease outbreaks.
World Wide Web URL: http://www.cdc.gov/travel

CNN Interactive

From breaking news to wire service stories, the CNN site gives you access to news and information almost as it happens. The site contains clickable headings such as WORLD, U.S., POLITICS, WEATHER, BUSINESS, SPORTS, SCI-TECH (science and technology), ENTERTAINMENT, BOOKS, TRAVEL, HEALTH, and others. There is even an option to customize the news you receive.
World Wide Web URL: http://www.cnn.com/

CNN-Sports Illustrated

For sports fans of all sorts, this site can give you minute-by-minute scores, recaps and feature stories, audio and video, and more. (I don't know if it carries the swimsuit issue.)
World Wide Web URL: http://sportsillustrated.cnn.com/

CNNFN-The Financial Network

This is the financial cousin of the CNN site and provides ample business news and information for even the most dedicated stock watcher.
World Wide Web URL: http://cnnfn.cnn.com/

CollegeBound Network

Another excellent site for students and parents facing the process of college selection, application, and matriculation.
World Wide Web URL: http://collegebound.net

Concierge.com

What a fun site! It includes content from Conde Nast Travel Guides . The site is basically divided into three sections: places, planning, play. You can search for information on a specific place. Under "Planning," are the "World Calendar of Events" and "Deal of the Week," a recommended travel deal. An especially handy item is the "All-in-One Sign Up for Airfare Bargains on the Net." This page has brought together registration for eight of the e-mail-notification saver fare bulletins (all reviewed by Conde Nast) including US Air, American, TWA, Continental, Iceland Air, Cathay-Pacific, Southwest, and Air Canada.
World Wide Web URL: http://www.concierge.com/

CondéNet

Here you can find features from the many Conde Nast magazines, including *The New Yorker, Travel and Leisure, Architectural Digest, Vanity Fair, Bon Appetit, Gourmet, Self, Women's Health and Fitness.*
World Wide Web URL: http://www.condenast.com

Consumer Reports

This is the on-line version of the popular *Consumer Reports.* The site offers all you would expect from the magazine along with seasonal or topical features.
World Wide Web URL: http://www.consumerreports.org/

eBAy On-line Auction

With 3 million items being auctioned at any one time, this is the busiest on-line auction. Browsing, registering, and bidding couldn't be easier. Multiple search functions and the ability to track those items you have bid on make it easy to get addicted. The system even sends you e-mail notices when you have been outbid or have won an item.
World Wide Web URL: http://www.ebay.com/

Education Unlimited

Have a teenager? This is the site that can give lots of information about colleges and universities. College ratings, application procedures, information about the SAT and ACT, financial aid, and more can be found at this portal to the Web.
World Wide Web URL: http://eunetwork.com

Epicurious Food

Recipes and content from *Bon Appetit* and *Gourmet* magazines. Filled with everything from etiquette to "victual reality" and of course recipes for everything from perfect gravy to a meatless Thanksgiving menu! Also includes restaurant reviews from all over the globe.
World Wide Web URL: http://www.epicurious.com/

Excite Travel

One of a number of similar sites, Excite Travel is Excite's travel agency offering hotel, airline, and other reservation services.
World Wide Web URL: http://travel.excite.com/

International Travelers Clinic

The Medical College of Wisconsin International Travelers Clinic located at Froedtert Hospital provides comprehensive preventive health care services for travelers planning trips abroad. The site provides lots of health information important for the international traveler.
World Wide Web URL: http://www.intmed.mcw.edu/travel.html

Lycos Maps

At this site you can type in the street or address you want to find and get a custom-drawn map. This site is great if you are traveling to unfamiliar places near or far. You can enter any two addresses and get directions, driving distance and time, and a map, all in a matter of seconds. If you want to get fancy, you can enter a telephone number and have the site tell you where the call came from.
World Wide Web URL: http://maps.lycos.com

The New York Times

News as well as classifieds, arts, restaurants, and more are here at the electronic version of "all the news that's fit...."
World Wide Web URL: http://www.nytimes.com

PC Quote.com

One of many services that can supply stock quotes and information.
World Wide Web URL: http://www.pcquote.com/

Public Broadcasting

In addition to what's on tonight, the site features wonderful information on science, technology, art, music, nature, analysis from the News Hour with Jim Lehrer, and an award-winning children's section, www.pbs.org/kids. Searchable listings of everything from current and recently shown television offerings, to listings of local stations and activities for children. News, learning resources, and PBS-branded merchandise are all here as well.
World Wide Web URL: http://www.pbs.org/

Reel.com

Reel.com was created to help you discover great new movies you'll love, and to let you buy and rent those movies. From new releases to kids video to old classics and hard-to-find films, this site is the video equivalent of the on-line bookstores. It has 100,000 movies for sale—seven times as large a selection as a

typical video superstore—and 35,000 movies for rent. The site includes the American Film Institute's top 100 films, previews, and reviews to help you make selections.
World Wide Web URL: http://www.reel.com/

SmartMoney.com

The SmartMoney site provides access to a number of financial planning tools and information resources.
World Wide Web URL: http://www.smartmoney.com

Time.com

This site is an interesting mixture of articles and features from the wide array of Time-Warner periodicals, including *Time, Money, Fortune, Mutual Funds, People, Entertainment Weekly*. Also links to Zagat's Restaurant Review on the Web and much more.
World Wide Web URL: http://www.time.com/time/index.html

The Washington Post

Here is a chance to follow what is being said in one of the country's most influential papers. The site includes features such as "Today's Edition" and "Yesterday's Edition" so when people are discussing something in the paper and you didn't have time to stop and buy it, you can go back to the site and look!
World Wide Web URL: http://www.washingtonpost.com

The Weather Channel

The Weather Channel home page provides weather information for anywhere in the world. This can be useful when planning trips to meetings. It also provides medically related information such as pollen maps and information about colds and flu.
World Wide Web URL: http://www.weather.com

United Parcel Service

The UPS site allows you to calculate transit times and track shipments on-line—helpful when you are expecting that package from eBay.
World Wide Web URL: http://www.ups.com/

USA Today

It is only logical that a paper that is composed and published almost exclusively by electronic means should be on the Web. The site offers the usual new and information, but is particularly strong in sports and weather information—a real help when traveling.

World Wide Web URL: http://www.usatoday.com

Walt Disney Company

This is the portal to almost limitless fun, adventure, resources, and trivia any Disney fan could want. Like sites presented by other entertainment companies such as Warner Brothers, Paramount, and others, you can find on-line movie trailers, contests, deck-top icons, sounds, screen savers, and merchandise.

World Wide Web URL: http://www.disney.go.com/park/homepage/today/ flash/index.html?clk=1004398

Whowhere?

A portal to a number of sites that can help you locate almost anyone in the United States.

World Wide Web URL: http://www.whowhere.lycos.com/

Other Sites of Interest

Center for the Easily Amused

Billed as the ultimate guide to wasting time on the Internet. Try checking out this site.

World Wide Web URL: http://www.amused.com/

Health Care Humor

A collection of medically related humor (good and groaners). Visitors are invited to submit their own humor.

World Wide Web URL: http://www.webcom.com/mdtaxes/humor.html

Managed Health Links

Managed Health Links is an on-line gateway to managed care Web sites on the Internet. Managed Health Links makes it easier to find managed care information on the Internet.
World Wide Web URL: http://www.managedhealthlinks.com/

Medic Alert

Information about the MedicAlert system.
World Wide Web URL: http://www.medicalert.org/

Glossary

10BaseT: A method of distributing Ethernet data short distances over ordinary telephone lines.

Address: The physical, or conceptional, location of information within the computer, usually used to refer to memory locations. In Internet parlance, the string of information (human or machine readable) that specifies the location of the information of interest and the computer upon which it is located.

ADSL: Asymmetric Digital Subscriber Line. A method of transmitting data at high speeds over telephone lines. In this system the speeds of transmission in one direction or the other may differ.

Alias: A name or placeholder for a file, application, destination, or grouping of information. A special recipient name for a group of Internet addresses.

Anonymous FTP: Computer site set to allow public retrieval of files using the login "anonymous."

Applet: A small computer program, written in the Java programming language, that is downloaded and run under the auspices of an Internet browser program.

Application: A group of instructions that tell the computer how to accomplish a task. This is usually a relatively complex set of instructions, that handle a variety of related tasks necessary to accomplish an overall type of task, such as word processing, making a graph, or playing music.

Archie: An information retrieval system for anonymous FTP sites.

Archive: A set of one or more files that have been compressed to save space or speed up transmission over the Internet. Many of these files have names that end in .zip, .sit depending on the compression program used to create the file.

ASCII: American Standard Code for Information Interchange. A computer code for expressing numerals, letters of the alphabet, and other symbols based on eight bits of binary code.

ASP: Either Active Server Page or Application Service Provider. Active Server Page is a scripting environment for Microsoft Internet Information Server in which you can combine HTML, scripts, and reusable ActiveX server components to create dynamic Web pages. An Application Service Provider is an Internet-based provider of application programs that reside on the provider's computer but are used by (loaned to) the Internet user or subscriber. In this service, the data may reside on your computer, but the application that uses the data remains on the server.

Attachment: One or more files that are sent along with an electronic mail message.

Audio board/ sound card: Some computers require the addition of an additional circuit board to play monophonic or stereophonic sounds. With such a card and a compact disc player, the computer may play music, or utilize sounds embedded within software programs. Many computers require a sound card to play music or transmit voice over the Internet.

Back door: A secret way into a computer or computer program that bypasses the normal security procedures.

Backbone: The basic communications link of a network.

Bandwidth: A measure of the amount of information that may be transmitted at a given time. Applied to the Internet in general, but may be applied to any method of information transmission. Often used in off-hand comments about the content of information, such as "It was a waste of bandwidth," to indicate wasteful or frivolous information.

Baud: This term, introduced in 1931 and named for the French inventor J. M. E. Baudot, is a measure of the speed of transmission of information. Originally applied to Teletype information, it is roughly equal to one character per second.

BBS: Bulletin Board System. Electronic bulletins board where messages may be read or posted for others to see.

Binary: Based on two alternatives, such as mathematical base 2. In this base, only two digits represent all numbers: 1 and 0. Like the base 10 that we use every day, position relative to the rightmost digit determines the exponential value of each digit. When summed the final valued is reached. In base 10 (B_{10}) the expression 123 is equivalent to 1 times 10^2, plus 2 times 10^1, plus 3 times 10^0. Since $10^2 = 100$, $10^1 = 10$, and $10^0 = 1$, this gives us $100 + 20 + 3 = 123$. In base 2 the same principle applies except that the base number used for each place is 2. Therefore, $1011_2 = 1$ times 2^3, plus 0 times 2^2, plus 1 times 2^1, plus 1 times 2^0 or $8 + 0 + 2 + 1 = 11_{10}$.

Bit: The smallest unit of information. A unit of information that may have two states (e.g., 1 or 0). This may represent any information that has two mutually exclusive conditions, such as true or false, on or off, light or dark, etc. In a binary string, it represents one digit. In computing, a bit is a single 1 or 0 stored in the computer.

Bookmark: An Internet address (URL) that is stored in a folder for future reference. In Netscape the file is called the bookmark file, while Internet Explorer calls the file favorites.

Bounce or **bounce back:** To have an electronic mail message returned as undeliverable. This may happen if you have a bad address or if the receiving party cannot receive mail at that time (e.g., server is off-line).

Browser: A computer program that acts as an intermediary or agent that requests and interprets information sent over the Internet.

Buss: The electronic highway that the computer uses to send information back and forth between the central processor, memory locations, special chips that perform special tasks such as a video generator, or the outside world by way of ports.

Byte: A collection of bits, usually in multiples of two, such as 4, 8, 16, or 32. This represents the width (in bits) of a computer "word." The larger the byte a computer can use, the more information that may be contained in a single word. A byte that is four bits wide can contain only 16 (2^4) possible combinations of 1s and 0s. By contrast, a 32-bit byte can contain over 4 million combinations (2^{32}).

Channel or **chat room:** One of several terms used for an area where Internet users may exchange live text messages. Channels and chat rooms often have themes that provide a common thread or topic of conversation. Some channels or chat rooms have a monitor to keep order, some do not.

Client: A computer that uses the services of another computer (a server).

Clock speed: A timing "clock" coordinates all of the activities of the computer. All activities take place as discrete steps that are kept in cadence by this clock. As a result, the faster the clock speed, the more instructions or activities the computer can accomplish in a give amount of time. Because of the amount of data transferred and manipulated during and Internet session, a computer with a fast clock speed is required.

Cookies: A small file left on your computer (in the hard drive) that saves information about you and your interaction with the distant computer Web site. This information may contain when you last visited, your shirt size, type of computer you use, or your preference in books. The next time you visit that Web site, it can retrieve the cookie and use the information to customize its interaction with you.

CPU: Central Processing Unit. This is the "thinker" that makes the computer function. This is the chip that interprets the software instructions, performs operation such as addition and subtraction, stores and requests information from memory, and makes logical decisions. It is this branching to various parts of a computer program based on conditions that could not be known at the time the program was written that makes computers so powerful. Like clock speed, the more powerful the CPU, the faster and easier Internet travel becomes.

Cursor: An indicator (flashing box, line, underline, arrow, or other image) displayed on the computer monitor that tells the user where the next action will take place.

Daemon: An automatic utility program that runs in the background of a computer. Often used to respond to requests for information or to handle incoming mail.

Digest: A collection of messages about a specific topic prepared by a mailing list moderator.

Disinter-mediation: The ability to directly connect two parties without the use of an intermediary. Examples include directly entering an order into a seller's computer system without a sales agent or distributor, and the obtaining information directly from a source that was previously available only through an intermediate agent.

Document: A body of data that may be interpreted by an application. This may be information about the look and content of a letter, how to draw a picture or graph on the screen, the contents of a spreadsheet, or any other body of data that an application may need to carry out its task. Generally these data are specific to a set of circumstances that the user has specified and are not required for the normal operation of the application. (See Resource.)

Domain name: Name of a computer system that is registered with the Internet. Can be made up of subdomains such as geographic or organizational subdomains.

Download: To obtain a file of data or a program from a remote computer.

DSL: Digital Subscriber Line. A high-speed form of telephone connection that is becoming more common in residential areas. Connections must be within a maximal limit of the telephone company's switching system (generally 3 miles). These connections require a special form of modem.

Dynamic rerouting: Ability of a network to direct communications around a damaged connection to still reach the intended recipient.

E-mail: Electronic mail.

Emoticons: Icons for indicating emotions (see Chapter 2, Table 2.7).

EPROM: Erasable programmable read-only memory. A type of ROM that may be altered by the user or machine but that retains the information when the power is removed. This is useful for storing some types of information, such as start-up preferences, security passwords, etc.

Ethernet: A fast local network originally developed by Xerox Corporation.

Eudora: A mail-handling program for either Windows or Macintosh computers.

FAQ: Frequently asked question(s).

File: Like a document, this is a collection of data. The term is less specific and may apply to a document, application, or other collection of related data.

Film recorder: Similar to a printer, this device uses instructions passed from the computer to draw information onto film using a very narrow beam of light, passed through one of three primary filters. Just as a printer "draws" a letter on the paper, film printers "draw" information onto film, which may then be developed to reveal the image.

Firewall: A combination of hardware and software used to keep unauthorized users from accessing part or all of a computer's files or connections.

Firewire: A proprietary (Macintosh) connection port for high-speed transmission of digital video data.

Flame: To post angry or insulting messages. This may lead to a flame war, or (fruitless) exchange.

Forum: Same as a Newsgroup.

FreeNet: A computer network that brings together the resources of a community or campus and is available free of charge.

Freeware: Software distributed at no cost. It cannot be sold or incorporated into other software, but may be freely distributed.

FTP: File Transfer Protocol. A set of specifications that support Internet file transfer.

Gateway: Computer system that acts as a point of access that allows information to move back and forth between networks. Often used when the networks involved use different protocols.

GIF: Graphics Interchange Format. A form of graphics file compression developed by CompuServe to be used for file transmission over the Web. These files are generally larger than files using the JPEG format.

Gigabyte: One billion bytes of data.

Gopher: A way of organizing and categorizing certain types of information on the Internet.

Graphics tablet: A type of information input device that uses a pen or other cursor devices on a special surface or tablet to draw, write, or select options. This type of input device is very commonly used for graphic arts and design work.

GUI: Graphic User Interface. The "desktop" metaphor used by Macintosh computers and the Windows series of operating systems. These interfaces use icons such as folders and sheets of paper to take the place of directories and data documents to facilitate use by those not familiar with the details of computer structure or function.

Hacker: A person that attempts, for fun or other purposes, to use unauthorized means to enter and use other computers. Generally applied to computer entry via the Internet.

Hardware: Physical computer equipment.

Header: Information placed at the start of an electronic mail message that assists with routing and the display of the message.

Hit(s): Visit(s) to a Web page over a period of time.

Home page: A Web page about a person or organization. Often used to mean the first screen of information that someone sees when accessing a Web site or opening a browser program.

Host: A synonym for any computer connected to the Internet, generally at a remote location.

HTML: Hypertext Markup Language. A computer language used to transmit information about the display of graphics, text, music, and other information. The language allows commands to be embedded that instruct the computer on what information is to be displayed, in what manner, and where that information may be found. The language allows references to information to take the place of the information itself, resulting in smaller files and faster information transfer. Most Web browsers interpret HTML instructions as part of the process of creating the Web page we see.

HTTP/HTTPS: HyperText Transfer Protocol. The way the World Wide Web transfers pages over the Internet. The additional "S" indicates an encrypted or secure transmission protocol.

Hyperlink: A word or phrase displayed in an Internet browser (or elsewhere) that will take the user to related information. In text, these are most often displayed in a different color, underlined, or both. When a graphic or icon is used as the starting point, the user's cursor will change to a hand when passed over the active link. In either case, a mouse click on the link will take the user to the related material.

Hypertext: Text that contains embedded links to other data.

Initialization string: A series of characters that is sent as commands to a modem that establish the settings to be used. The exact commands required will be contained in the modem's user manual.

Internet: The name for a group of worldwide computer-based information resources connected together.

InterNIC: Internet Network Information Center. A central repository of information about the Internet and site where domain names may be registered. (**http://www.internic.net**)

I/O device: Input/output device, or a device that allows communications between the user and the computer. It may take many forms: a keyboard, display screen, printer, scanner, modem, film recorder, or mass storage device such as a hard, floppy, or compact disc drive. Some of these communicate in only one direction, while others are capable of two-way communication. Collectively, many of these devices are referred to as peripheral devices. The most common I/O devices involved in using the Internet are modems or network interface cards.

ISDN: Integrated Services Digital Network. A very high-speed connection (usually a dedicated telephone line) used to link computers to the Internet or to connect one computer to another.

ISP: Internet Service Provider. A third-party provider that supplies access and temporary Internet addresses to users by way of dial-up modem connections. In many cases, the provider also supplies additional services such as e-mail accounts, databases, chat rooms, etc.

Java: A programming language that allows small applications to be transmitted across the Internet and run independently of the computer platform used. These programs generally perform small tasks related to the display of information in Web browsers.

Jazz disk: A trade-named removable disk based on technology introduced by Iomega, which can store approximately 1 gigabyte of information. The term, like Kleenex and Xerox, has become generalized to refer to high-capacity small diskettes.

Joystick: A pointing device based on the two-dimensional motions of a control stick. Common in the early days of computing and in game playing, now relegated mainly to the world of video games.

JPEG: Joint Photographic Expert Group. Compression standard used to format pictorial information. Files formatted using this standard usually have names that end in **.jpg** or **.jpeg**. Usually pronounced "JAY-peg."

Jughead: An information retrieval system for a specific Gopher site.

Keystroke logger: A program that automatically keeps a file of everything that is typed from the keyboard.

Link: A hypertext pointer to another file or Web site that may be invoked by pointing and clicking on the appropriate portion of the displayed Web page. The term also refers to the text-based reference to the URL provided in the Web page instructions themselves.

Listserv: Listserver, the most common computerized mailing list administration program.

Login ID: Unique identifying character string assigned to a user of a computer system.

Luddite: A person who believes that the progress brought by machines is dangerous to the public good.

Lurk or lurking: Listening in on a mailing list or newsgroup discussion without replying.

Lynx: A text-based Web browser program.

Mail server: A computer that provides electronic mail services.

Mailbot: A computer program that automatically sends or answers electronic mail.

Mailing list: A collection of Internet addresses that facilitates an electronic discussion group.

Mass storage device: One of several types of devices that store large amounts of data in the form of files. Most common are hard disk and floppy disk drives. Compact disk players that can read computer files stored on CD-ROM disks also come under this heading. Internet surfing requires a large amount of storage space for both intermediate files used by the Web browser to display each page and by the audio, video, and picture files often transferred and stored by the user.

Megabyte: One million bytes.

Memory: A nonspecific term for the area in which information is stored. The term may be applied to the working memory of the computer, such as RAM, ROM, etc., or to mass storage devices such as disk drives.

MIDI: Musical Instrument Digital Interface. A protocol for transmitting music as a series of commands (notes) rather than as the sounds themselves, allowing the receiving device to play them in their own way. Many electronic instruments can sent or receive MIDI information.

MIME: Multipurpose Internet Mail Extension. A system used to send text, pictures, programs, and other nontext information as a part of electronic mail.

Mirror: One or more computers that share (mirror) the same information so that the load on popular sites may be spread out to improve access speed. In some systems, a mirror site may be selected automatically and the user is unaware of its use; in others, users may choose the mirror site they wish to use.

Modem: Derived from the terms "modulate" and "demodulate," a modem uses telephone or other communications routes to transmit data. The speed and protocol by which this is done varies, but shares the common feature of converting digital information into a varying tone that may be carried by the communications path and interpreted by the receiving modem, which converts the tone back into digital information.

Mosaic: A Windows-based Web browser program that was the predecessor of most of the advanced browsers in use today.

Mouse: A type of pointing device that moves on the physical desktop to move a cursor on the computer screen. The mouse usually has one or more buttons or switches with which to indicate choices.

MP3: Motion Picture Experts Group-1, Audio Layer-3. A format for compressing sound into small computer files.

MPEG: Motion Picture Experts Group. A standard (now in its fourth iteration) for how video information is compressed and transmitted.

Multimedia: An overused term for anything that uses more than one media, such as sound, images, movies, and the like. The term is not specific and may be applied to almost any type of software product.

Netscape: A Web browser program available for both Macintosh and PC (IBM compatible) computers.

Network: Two or more computers connected together so that information can move between them.

Newbie: A newcomer to the Internet, just a step up from clueless newbie.

Newsgroup: A collecting site for messages about a specific theme.

Newsreaders: Programs used to access a newsgroup, such as rn, tn, nn, and tin.

Node: A computer (host or server) on the Internet.

OCR: Optical Character Reader. A type of scanner and software that allow a printed page to be "read" into the computer and interpreted as a string of characters rather than an image.

Packet: A chunk of information traveling as a bundle over the Internet. The packet contains information about its origin and destination, file type and size, and additional information about confirmation of receipt, etc.

Parallel port: A pathway for information transfer in which the data are moved as a byte or word over a series of wires that simultaneously have a sequence of 1's and 0's.

Password: String of characters secretly chosen to verify that you are the valid user connected with a specific user ID.

PCMCIA/PCI: Personal Computer Memory Card International Association/ Peripheral Component Interconnect. First developed as a standard for add-on memory for portable and palm-top computers, this now refers to a standard that allows chip-based peripheral components to be plugged directly into a special port to provide special functions such as FAX, modems, or memory. These are mainly found on newer portable machines.

PDA: Personal Digital Assistant. A palm-top computer or other microprocessor-based hand-held devices that perform multiple functions. As cell phone technology evolves, these devices may join this group.

PDF: Portable Document Format. This format is used to contain complex documents with graphs, images, and special text that cannot be presented easily through the typical Web browser. The creator of this file format, Adobe Systems, offers a free viewer (Adobe Acrobat Reader) to view any PDF file. There are versions for most operating systems.

PIM: Personal Information Manager. A palm-top computer or Internet-based system of organizing appointments, reminders, names, addresses, and other similar information. Information may be displayed in a number of formats with customized reminders. Internet-based systems may be configured to automatically seek information of this type to be added to your personal files, thus acting as a (partially) intelligent agent.

Pixel: Picture element. The smallest unit used to make a picture on the monitor screen or printer output. The smaller the pixel, the more detailed the picture; the more pixels, the larger the image.

Plug-in: A small computer program that is added to another (usually your browser program) that adds special functionality or a special type of information such as music or video.

Pointing device: Any one of several types of devices used to move a cursor on the computer display. Common types are the mouse, track ball, trackpad, joystick, or graphics tablet.

POP: Point of Presence. Literally, a connection to the Internet. Generally refers to an Internet service provider (ISP) that provides access to the Internet by temporarily assigning an Internet address from a group owned by the provider.

Port: A pathway in and out of the physical box that contains the computer. This path may transfer raw information, or information that has already been processed into a different form, such as a telephone or video signal.

PPP: Point-to-Point Protocol. A protocol that allows the use of someone else's Internet presence on a temporary basis. Internet service providers allow a user to connect to the Internet using this protocol.

Printer: Any device that converts computer information and places it on a printed page. This may be accomplished by the use of a sophisticated typewriter-like device (daisy-wheel printer), a group of small pins that draw letters and images as a set of finely spaced dots (dot-matrix printer), sprayed small droplets of ink ("jet" printers), heated elements that transfer wax (thermal transfer), or drawing the image onto a copier-like drum using a small beam of light ("laser" printers). Speed, quality, and the possibility of color printing vary with the technology used.

Protocol: Agreed-upon rules for communications between devices (generally computers, modems, or fax machines). These include signals that mean "start," "stop," "got it," "send again," "all done," etc.

Push technology: Methods that allow information posted on a Web site to be sent automatically to others without waiting for them to request it. This is somewhat analogous to broadcasting the information, but unlike broadcasting, the sender is assured the information will be received.

QuickTime: A video file format widely used on the Internet. Originally developed by Apple Computer but available for all platforms.

RAM: Random Access Memory. This is the memory that may be used by the user and software to store information on a temporary basis. Any location may be addressed at any time. This memory is "volatile" and the information stored there will be lost if the power is lost or if some other information is placed in the same location.

Resource: A set of data, often stored in the same location as the application itself, that is used by the application to accomplish a specific part of its work. Resources may be icons, sounds, images, information, or portions of a dialog directed toward the user. This information is generally only for the use of the application, and may not be addressed or used by the user under normal circumstances.

ROM: Read-Only Memory. This is memory that contains information used by the computer operating system that is independent of the software program that is running. This information is placed there by the computer designers and is permanently place into memory at the time the chips are manufactured. This memory is not lost when the power is turned off, allowing this type of memory to help in the start-up process.

Router: A computer that connects two or more networks.

Scanner: This device is used to convert physical materials into computer renderings. This may be in the form of a picture "copied" from a printed source, the image of a printed page, or through the use of special software, a transcript of the printed page that may be manipulated in a word processing program.

SCSI: Small Computer Serial Interface ("skuzzy"). This is a high-speed pathway for communicating between the computer and special input-output devices, most notably memory storage devices such as hard disks, CD-ROM drives, input devices such as scanners, and the like.

Search engine: A program used to find information on the World Wide Web.

Secure socket: A form of encryption used when transmitting and receiving data.

Serial port: A pathway for information transfer in which the data are moved as a series of 1's and 0's. This is the most common point of connection for a modem.

Server: A general term for any computer that supplies information to other computers. The term may also be applied to the software the facilitates the transfer.

Shareware: Computer programs that are widely distributed on the honor system. You may try the program at no charge, but it is understood that you will send a user or registration fee if you decide to keep and use the program.

SIMM/DIMM: Single In-line Memory Module/Dual In-line Memory Module. A small, single- or double-sided circuit card that may be inserted into a computer to provide additional RAM.

SLIP: Serial Line Internet Protocol. A protocol that allows the use of someone else's Internet presence on a temporary basis. Internet service providers allow a user to connect to the Internet using this protocol.

SMTP: Simple Mail Transfer Protocol. The system used to pass mail from one Internet computer to another.

Socket: The logical "port" used by one computer program to connect to another program running on the Internet.

Software: The group of instructions that the computer uses to carry out one or more tasks.

Spam: The act of sending unrequested electronic mail. Generally restricted to mass-mailing types of mail or newsgroup postings. Also, a proprietary meat product from Hormel, Inc.

Surf: To wander around sites on the World Wide Web looking for interesting material.

TCP/IP: Transmission Control Protocol/Internet Protocol

Telnet: A program used to connect to a remote computer.

Terminal emulation connection: The process that allows your computer screen and keyboard to control a remote computer.

Trackball: A pointing device that moves the computer cursor based on the movements of an upturned ball, somewhat analogous to an overturned mouse.

Trackpad: A pointing device that senses the movement of a finger over its surface.

Trojan horse: A program or message that contains a virus or worm inside.

Upload: To move a file of data or a program to a remote computer.

URL: Uniform Resource Locator. A standardized method for referencing an item on the World Wide Web, including a complete description and its location.

USB: Universal Serial Bus. A high-speed connection found on the newer computers that is used to connect to other devices.

Usenet: User's Network, made up of all machines that receive network newsgroups.

User ID: User identification, synonymous with login ID.

Veronica: An information retrieval system for Gopher sites.

Video card: Many computers require a separate card (electronic circuit board) to produce the video signal sent to the monitor. This card often contains its own dedicated memory (VRAM) to allow more colors, higher resolution, or faster displays.

Virtual memory: A technique that allows space on a hard disk to act as if it were part of the computer's active (RAM) memory.

Virus: Small computer programs that "infect" a computer of files by starting its own operation without the permission or knowledge of the operator. These programs make copies of themselves, allowing them to infect other computers. Viruses vary from those that put a surprise message on the monitor, to those that will erase data or corrupt files. A number of commercial products exist to help identify, remove, or "immunize" against viruses. The use of specialized languages that has made Internet browsers and other tools so powerful (such as Applets and Java Scripts) now opens the possibility of viral transmission across the Internet.

VRML: A language used to build virtual reality pages on the World Wide Web.

WAIS: Wide Area Information Servers. A way of categorizing and organizing certain types of information on the Internet.

War dialer: A program that is used to dial a series of telephone numbers. Often used by hackers to look for computer modems.

WAV file: A format for transmitting sound files. File names generally end with **.wav**.

Web browser: An information retrieval program for the World Wide Web that can interpret and display hypertext documents.

WebTV: A method of connecting to the Internet using television cables to carry the signal and the user's home television to display the information.

World Wide Web (WWW): A hypermedia-based system that lets users browse through information stored in different formats.

Worm: A program that is similar to a virus in that it is an uninvited program that "lives" inside your computer and does damage. Worms do damage to computer files by moving through memory (active or storage) destroying what is stored there.

WORM: Write Once, Read Many. One of several types of storage systems, generally in the compact disk format, that allow information to be stored, but cannot be altered once the storage has taken place. This type of storage is attractive for applications where a record of all changes made must be maintained. An example might be patient records, where future additions or alterations must be documented along with the original information.

WYSWYG: "What you see is what you get." Refers to print and other documents that appear on the computer display in the same way that they will appear when printed to paper or a film recorder.

XML: Extensible Markup Language. A set of extensions to the HTML language that expand functionality.

Zip disk: A trade-named removable disk based on technology introduced by Iomega, which can store approximately 100 megabytes of information. The term, like Kleenex and Xerox, has become generalized to refer to high-capacity small diskettes.

Index